MIKEL A. ROTHENBERG, MD

Laboratory Tests Made Easy

A PLAIN ENGLISH APPROACH

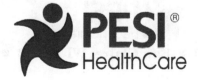

For information on this and other PESI HealthCare manuals
and audio recordings, please call **800-843-7763**
or visit our website: **www.pesihealthcare.com**

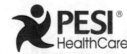

200 Spring Street, P.O. Box 900 ■ **Eau Claire, WI 54702** ■ **www.pesihealthcare.com**

OBJECTIVES

After completing this text, the learner will be able to:

1.   List three major reasons to obtain laboratory tests.

2.   Define the terms: specificity, sensitivity, positive predictive value, negative predictive value.

3.   Explain and discuss the reasoning behind the statement: "Normal tests do not mean a normal patient."

4.   Describe and explain how to use the Diagnostic Triangle.

5.   List the two most common causes of laboratory abnormalities.

6.   List the four most common drugs that affect laboratory values.

7.   For the following laboratory tests, describe at least two conditions that may explain abnormalities in each test:

- WBC
- H/H (Hgb/Hct)
- Platelet count
- Urinalysis
- Sodium
- Potassium
- Chloride
- Calcium
- Phosphorus
- Magnesium
- Blood sugar (glucose)
- BUN and creatinine
- Uric acid
- Liver function tests
- Thyroid function tests

8.   Discuss the role of laboratory tests in the diagnosis of the following diseases:

- Hepatitis A
- Hepatitis B
- Hepatitis C
- Hepatitis D

9. Describe and explain the role of each of the following tests in the diagnosis of HIV infection and AIDS:

- HIV antibody test
- CD4$^+$ lymphocyte levels
- CD8$^+$ lymphocyte levels
- Plasma HIV RNA (viral load)
- HIV drug resistance testing

10. Describe and utilize the "three question approach" to interpret a set of arterial blood gases.

11. Describe the role of and potential limitations of cardiac enzyme tests in acute myocardial infarction and acute coronary syndromes.

12. Explain the role of and potential limitations to the brain natriuretic protein (BNP) test in a patient presenting with shortness of breath.

13. Explain the difference in accuracy between non-β-HCG specific urine pregnancy tests and serum pregnancy tests.

14. For the following laboratory tests, describe at least two conditions that may explain abnormalities in each test:

- PT
- INR
- PTT

15. Describe the clinical implications of the following laboratory tests:

- Total cholesterol
- LDL-C
- HDL-C
- Triglycerides
- hs CRP

16. Explain the role of blood alcohol and drug screens as medical tests.

17. Describe the role of serum lipase and amylase measurements in the diagnostic work-up of a patient with abdominal pain.

18.   Describe three commonly performed microbiology tests.

19.   What is the clinical role of the following tests in diagnosis?

- Prostate specific antigen (PSA)
- Carcinoembryonic antigen (CEA)
- BRC gene tests
- HER-2 gene tests

LABORATORY TESTS MADE EASY – A PLAIN ENGLISH APPROACH
MIKEL A. ROTHENBERG, M.D.
2005

TABLE OF CONTENTS

REFERENCES

INDEX

CHAPTER 1 – INTRODUCTION
     THE "WHY" OF LABORATORY TESTS
     WHY ALL THE DIFFERENT TUBES?
     STATISTICS OF LAB TESTS
     PERILS AND PITFALLS OF LABORATORY TESTING
     MEDICAL DECISION MAKING – THE EASY WAY
     GENERAL APPROACH TO LAB STUDIES
     HOW TO USE THIS BOOK

CHAPTER 1 – INTRODUCTION

Laboratory tests are a part of just about all medical and surgical work-ups. It is imperative that all members of the health care team have a baseline understanding of these tests. A basic understanding of the different types of lab tests, their role in medical decision making, and an ability to recognize and deal promptly with abnormal values is an essential skill for all health care professionals. This text provides all the necessary information you'll need to do this in a medically proper fashion. I've also included "enrichment" information for those of you who want more details, references included! See "How to Use This Book," below, for details on how to apply the material herein to your day to day practice.

THE "WHY" OF LABORATORY TESTS

Laboratory tests are ordered for a variety of different reasons. All, when utilized properly, play an important role in the health care system. There are three major reasons to obtain laboratory tests:

- Screening – diagnosis of disease in an apparently healthy population. These types of tests are performed in healthy people to determine if they have a disease that is not clinically obvious. A example would be a fasting lipid profile in a person with no evidence of blood lipid abnormalities. Another is a fasting blood sugar in an obese patient who is over 40, but without any signs or symptoms of diabetes mellitus.

- Diagnosis – obtained to help detect the presence of a given condition (e.g., elevated blood sugar may indicate diabetes mellitus). It is important to remember that lab tests form only a part of our diagnostic armamentarium. Clinicians must use all available information (e.g., history, physical, x-ray, lab, etc.) to formulate a diagnosis – "tests don't make diagnoses, people do." (One of my favorite clinical philosophies!)

- Monitoring – serum levels of drugs; antibiotics, asthma drugs (theophylline preparations), anticoagulants. These tests allow us to follow the serum levels of medications and correlate these with the patient's clinical response.

WHY ALL THE DIFFERENT TUBES?

One of the questions patients inevitably ask us is, "Why do you need so much blood?" They usually wonder about this because the lab typically draws more than one tube. The answer is simple – different lab tests require that the blood be prepared in different ways. Each type of tube is made in a special way to best prepare that portion of the blood for a particular test. The details of all available types of tubes are beyond the scope of this discussion. Common "colored tubes" (based on the color of the stopper on the top) include:

- "Red top" (empty tube) – electrolytes, liver function tests, cardiac enzymes

- "Purple top" (contains EDTA, an anticoagulant) – complete blood count

- "Blue top" (contains sodium citrate; binds to calcium and prevents blood clotting) – protime (PT), partial thromboplastin time (PTT), international normalized ratio (INR)

- "Yellow top" – blood cultures

STATISTICS OF LAB TESTS

There are specific formulas to calculate the parameters discussed below. These are important in research, but of little value in clinical practice. The bottom line terms, however, as defined "functionally" below, are helpful:

- Specificity – number of true positive results; the more specific a test, the more likely a positive result truly indicates an abnormality. I think of the specificity as representing the false positive rate (note the "p" in both specificity and in false-positive) – a test that is highly specific (i.e., 98% specificity) has a *low* false positive rate (i.e., 2% false positives). Low specificity (i.e., 60%), on the other hand, means there is a *high* false positive rate (i.e., 40%).

- Sensitivity – number of true negatives; the more sensitive a test, the more likely a negative result truly indicates *absence* of an abnormality. I think of the sensitivity as representing the false negative rate (note the "n" in both sensitivity and in false-negative) – a test that is highly sensitive (i.e., 98% sensitivity) has a *low* false negative rate (i.e., 2% false negatives). Low sensitivity (i.e., 60%), on the other hand, means there is a *high* false negative rate (i.e., 40%).

- Positive predictive value – the chances that a given test result indicate the *presence* of a condition or disease.

- Negative predictive value – the chances that a given test result indicate the *absence* of a condition or disease

PERILS AND PITFALLS OF LABORATORY TESTING

As a rule, laboratory testing is straight forward. There are a couple of rules to keep in mind that will avoid confusion:

- Normal values vary between labs – depending on the method that a particular laboratory uses for a test, the normal values between labs may vary markedly. Though the values for many common tests (e.g., serum electrolytes) are universally similar, some vary widely from area to area (e.g., CPK, pO_2) and country to country (e.g., blood sugar). The good news is that virtually every laboratory you'll deal with provides the normal range in their laboratory, along with the patient result. Because of differences in normal values between laboratories, it is sometimes difficult to compare lab work done in several institutions. In these cases, it's easiest to just use "normal," "low," or "high" rather than the absolute values when making comparisons.

- Normal test not mean "normal" patient – though intuitively obvious to all of us, this statement bears remembering. Most tests we do, not just laboratory ones, are most helpful when they *confirm* what we already suspect – they are considerably less helpful in "ruling out" many conditions. For example, an elevated CPK-MB in a patient with two hours of crushing, substernal chest pain, is compatible with acute myocardial infarction (MI). On the other hand, a normal CPK-MB, especially when obtained within the first four hours of chest pain onset, does little to "rule out" an MI.

MEDICAL DECISION MAKING – THE EASY WAY

The Diagnostic Triangle, illustrated in **Figure 1-1**, is a summary of medical decision making. Originally termed the "triangulation approach" to clinical diagnosis and understanding, it is useful in *all* areas of medicine, not just in evaluating laboratory tests. There are three parts to the triangle:

1. Findings – this part describes the objective results (e.g., the white cell count [WBC], a heart murmur, 6 mm of ST-segment elevation on an EKG, a right middle lobe infiltrate on a chest x-ray). We accumulate sets of findings via our patient work-up.

2. Possible explanations for the findings – the second part of the "triangulation approach" is a right-brain process emphasizing "brainstorming" possible reasons for or causes of the described findings. The beauty of this system is that it is very patient safe and friendly – by emphasizing differential diagnosis, it encourages the clinician to consider, even though briefly at times, several diagnostic possibilities. Many can be excluded ("ruled out") in the next step (see below). So, possible explanations for an elevated WBC count might include: infection, dehydration, demargination of white blood cells (detaching from blood vessel walls) due to stress, drug effect (e.g., epinephrine), or leukemia.

3. Additional information – using additional information (e.g., history, physical, other tests, your previous knowledge, "gut" feelings [yes, I think that is very important!]) to narrow down the above list of "possibilities," to the most likely "probabilities," or working differential diagnosis. So, if the patient had a productive cough, fever, and physical signs of lung consolidation, the most likely explanations for an elevated WBC count would be infection and dehydration. See how the additional information allowed us to "narrow down" the possibilities. So, our differential diagnosis would be infection and dehydration. Remember, that the two are not necessarily mutually exclusive.

Thus, the triangulation system involves first listing the findings, then brainstorming possible explanations, and finally, narrowing these down to the most probable causes – the differential diagnosis

And, now the most important point – I call it the "medical national flower, the hedge!" Most of us are used to seeing a statement at the bottom of an x-ray report saying something alone the lines of "suggest clinical correlation," right? What the radiologist is really telling us is that his or her reading, despite the fact that he or she is a doctor, is no more than a test result. And people, not tests, make diagnoses. I urge clinicians to assume that a similar disclaimer is subconsciously attached to *any* set of findings that we deal with – history, physical, lab tests, diagnostic tests, etc. People, not tests, make diagnoses!

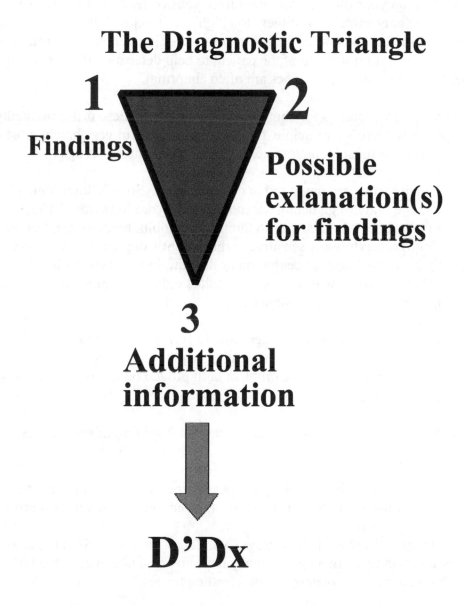

The Diagnostic Triangle

1

Findings

2

Possible exlanation(s) for findings

3

Additional information

D'Dx

Figure 1-1 – The Diagnostic Triangle helps frame medical diagnostic thinking by moving from findings, to possible explanations (possibilities), to a reasonable differential diagnosis (probabilities).

GENERAL APPROACH TO LAB STUDIES

Many laboratory tests are reported in terms of concentrations – cells per cubic milliliter, milligrams per deciliter, and such. A simple, yet helpful way to use this fact (assuming the parameter you're looking at is reported as a concentration) follows.

There are really only three possible results – normal, too high, or too low – agreed? Now, I've already said that a normal test, by itself, doesn't necessarily mean a normal patient – you'll have to make that part of the decision on your own (or with help from your colleagues, but *not* just from the lab work). As a rule though, if the concentration is either "too high" or "too low," the result is generally abnormal. So the first part of looking at the lab results is determining if they are in the normal range or not. Incorporate your clinical impression of the patient to help determine if "normal" is *really* normal or not. Then assume that "low" or "high" values are often abnormal.

There are lots of different causes for abnormal lab values, and these differ markedly, depending on the test you're looking at. Here's a principle, however, that comes in very handy most of the time – the two most common causes of most laboratory abnormalities are fluids or drugs . . .

Remember, most lab results are measured in concentrations. So it follows logically that any abnormality in fluid balance in the body (e.g., hemoconcentration, dehydration) would affect the measured *concentration* of substances (e.g., serum sodium, hemoglobin, hematocrit). Certain laboratory values (e.g., serum sodium) are extremely sensitive to the patient's degree of hydration and are clinically useful in helping diagnose hemoconcentration or dehydration. Others are less helpful (e.g., serum potassium). The bottom line – whenever a lab result is either "too high" or "too low," always consider some type of fluid imbalance as a possible cause.

Drugs should always be the second consideration. In fact, I've coined the term "Medicineheimer's Disease" meaning that if a patient is on medications and has a problem, one or more of the medications is contributing to or responsible for the problem until proven otherwise! And, this doesn't just apply to laboratory problems.

Regarding laboratory abnormalities, the most common drugs that affect the most significant laboratory tests are:

- Oxygen – other than the obvious (e.g., pO_2), hypoxia leads to increased erythropoietin production by the kidneys. This increases the hemoglobin and hematocrit values.

- Nonsteroidal anti-inflammatory drugs (NSAIDs) – various NSAIDs can affect liver and/or kidney function tests. In addition, many have an anti-platelet effect, which can affect coagulation tests (e.g., platelet count, bleeding time)

- Antibiotics – some antibiotics can precipitate hemolytic anemia (e.g., sulfa drugs) while other affect coagulation

- Diuretics – these can result in electrolyte imbalances (e.g., hypokalemia), as well as fluid balance abnormalities (e.g., dehydration) that, as noted above, commonly affect laboratory results.

Of course, *any* drug can conceivably lead to *any* abnormality in a given patient. So, the general rule when seeing a laboratory abnormality is to always consider early on either fluids or drugs as a potential cause.

HOW TO USE THIS BOOK

With a few exceptions, the organization of this book from chapter to chapter, is identical. The purpose is to allow you, the health care provider, to rapidly access *need to know* information regarding any particular lab test in the easiest possible fashion. I've also provided additional details, for those of you who are interested, interspersed through the text and at the end of some sections.

The general pattern of organization for each lab test is as follows:

- Parameters measured – a list of what tests are commonly obtained as part of any given "test."

- Test in a "nutshell" – a terse discussion of what the test covers, including why it may be ordered.

- Normal values – where available, typical normal values for laboratories in the United States and Canada have been summarized; remember, normals vary from hospital to hospital.

- Panic values – levels that most laboratory experts consider "potentially life-threatening." The laboratory generally contacts the provider, hospital floor, etc. immediately when a value in this range is noted. Generally, if the recipient of this information is not the ordering provider (e.g., physician, physician assistant, nurse practitioner), the person who first receives the "message" from the lab should immediately contact the provider. (*Note*: there may be other less "life-threatening" results that need to be given to the primary provider as soon as possible; however, these vary from case to case. The best way to deal with this situation is for the primary care provider to include, with standard orders, a list stating something like: "Contact me when: . . .").

- Results in a "nutshell" – the major causes of abnormalities in the measured parameter(s). Most of these are summarized in tabular form. This makes it easier for you to rapidly find the information you need and apply it immediately in your practice.

The above five sections are designed for rapid reference and review. This is where to look when you need the right answers, and need them right away.

- Test details – more specific information on each test. Though important, information in this section is better used when you have a few minutes to sit down and read it over at a more leisurely pace.

Depending on the test, I have included additional material that may be of interest to you. Much of this "enrichment" material is detailed, including references. I have marked this information for you: *(enrichment)*. In this fashion, readers of all levels of interest and experience can benefit from the book If you just need to "nitty gritty," use the first five sections detailed above; then read some of the "details" when you can. However, if you're interested in more details on the tests, including the pathophysiology of abnormalities, clinical treatment, and up-to-date research, it's in the "essays" interspersed throughout.

- Case studies – I've included several case studies in the last chapter (Chapter 13 – Case Studies) They are presented in the "programmed learning" form where we cover little pieces of information, topic by topic. Within the discussions, I have also interspersed some "enrichment" information that is not discussed in the body of the text. These are primarily to help you understand the use of various laboratory tests – I have deliberately excluded some information that you may normally have in a real clinical situation. Remember that people, *not* tests make diagnoses

CHAPTER 2 – THE COMPLETE BLOOD COUNT (CBC)

PARAMETERS MEASURED
THE TEST IN A "NUTSHELL"
NORMAL VALUES
PANIC VALUES
RESULTS IN A "NUTSHELL"
EMBRYOLOGICAL DEVELOPMENT
TYPES OF CELLS
RED CELL DISORDERS – ANEMIA AND POLYCYTHEMIA
WHITE CELL DISORDERS
PLATELET DISORDERS

CHAPTER 2 – THE COMPLETE BLOOD COUNT (CBC)

The **CBC**, or **complete blood count** determines the general composition of all the formed elements of the blood. It's helpful in numerous conditions especially infection and bleeding.

- **Parameters measured:**　　　WBC, differential, platelet count, Hgb, Hct (often referred together as H/H), MCV, MCH, MCHC

- **The test in a "nutshell":**　　Directly determines the numbers of white cells (WBC count) and their subtypes (differential count); the numbers of platelets (platelet count); and indirectly, the numbers of red cells (hemoglobin, hematocrit) and their size (MCV, MCH, MCHC). Morphology is evaluated by the **peripheral blood smear.** Commonly ordered to evaluate infection, weakness (anemia), bleeding.

- **Normal values:**

Adult	WBC X 10³	RBC X 10⁶	Hb g/dl	Hct (%)	MCV (fl)	MCH pg	MCHC g/dl	Plts 10³
Male	5.0-10.0	4.5-5.5	14.0-17.4	42-52	84-96	28-34	32-36	140-
Female	5.0-10.0	4.0-5.0	12.0-16.0	36-48	84-96	28-34	32-36	140-

PANIC VALUES!!

WBC < 500 or > 30,000

Hct < 20% (heart failure) or > 60% (spontaneous clotting)

Hgb < 5 g/dl or > 20 g/dl

Platelet count < 20,000 or > 1,000,000

- **Results in a "nutshell":**

PARAMETER	CAUSES OF ELEVATIONS	CAUSES OF DECREASES
WBC	infection, leukemia, demargination (stress, epinephrine)	leukemia, AIDS, viral infection, bone marrow suppression (drugs, toxins)
PLATELET COUNT	tumors (paraneoplastic syndromes), connective tissue disease (SLE), dehydration, polycythemia vera	leukemia, AIDS, bone marrow suppression (drugs, toxins)
H/H	polycythemia vera, COPD (chronic hypoxia), high altitude living	leukemia, AIDS, bone marrow suppression (drugs, toxins)

- **Embryological development** of the cell lines and hematopoiesis – there is a common precursor for all cell lines. This differentiates into the white cell, red cell, and platelet lines of development.

- **Types of cells (formed elements)**

There are three types of cells or formed elements in the peripheral blood: white blood cells, platelets, and red blood cells.

1. **White blood cells (WBC)** – fight against infection and foreign materials in the body

   ▸ **WBC count** – the total number of white blood cells per cc of blood; this is also referred to as the "total white count," by some providers.

   ▸ **Differential** – an enumeration of the different kinds of WBCs as a percentage of the total number of cells counted. There are two general types of WBCs – those that contain microscopic granules (granulocytes) and those that don't (agranulocytes). The different types are summarized in the table below.

   ▸ **WBC morphology** (size and shape) – if abnormal on the peripheral blood smear, a comment may appear in the report.

Type of cell (granulocytes shaded)	Normal range (%)	Combats:	Comment
Band	1-3	Pyogenic infections	Immature WBC; increased with acute infection (shift to the left); decreased with liver disease, megaloblastic anemia, some drugs and allergies (shift to the right)
Seg	50-62	Pyogenic infections	Primarily rely on phagocytosis; release enzymes and endogenous pyrogens
Eosinophil	1-4	Allergic disorders; parasitic infections	Ingest antigen-antibody complexes; active early in allergic reactions; respond in later stages of inflammation; circadian rhythm (lowest in the AM)
Basophil	0-1	Parasitic infections; tumors (associated with)	Phagocytosis; also contain heparin, histamines, and serotonin
Monocyte	0-5	Severe infections	Phagocytosis; reversibly transform with histiocytes (tissue macrophages)
Lymphocyte	25-45	Viral infections (measles, rubella, chickenpox, infectious mononucleosis)	Migrate to site of infection

[NOTE: a "shift to the left" means that the number of bands is increased, usually due to an acute infection. There is no such thing as a "shift to the right."]

2.   **Platelets** – major line of defense against bleeding from small holes in vessels, forming a "hemostatic plug."

> ▸   **Platelet count** – number of platelets per cc of blood

> ▸   **Platelet morphology and estimate** on peripheral smear – labs report when the number of platelets on the peripheral blood smear appears low. Abnormal platelet size and shape is unusual, but will be noted if present.

> ▸   **Bleeding time** – not part of routine CBC; measures platelet function but is subjective and not always used.

3.   **Red blood cells (RBC)** – transport oxygen to cells and carbon dioxide to the lungs.

> ▸   **RBC count** (rarely used by itself) – the number of red blood cells per cc of blood

> ▸   **Hemoglobin** (Hg or hgb) – oxygen-carrying protein in RBCs (gm/dl blood). Also serves as an ECF (extracellular fluid) buffer

> ▸   **Hematocrit** (Hct) – the packed cell volume of RBCs, expressed as a percentage of the total blood volume.

> ▸   **MCH** – mean corpuscular hemoglobin (MCH = hgb/RBC; picograms); measure of the amount of hgb per cell; essentially the same as MCV since hgb and hct are interrelated (hgb X 3 = hct).

> ▸   **MCHC** – mean corpuscular hemoglobin concentration (MCHC = hgb/hct; grams/100 ml RBCs); measure of the concentration (chromicity) of hgb in each RBC. Thus, RBCs may contain the normal hgb concentration (**normochromic**), less than normal (**hypochromic**), or greater than normal (**hyperchromic**).

> ▸   **MCV** – mean corpuscular volume (MCV = hct/RBC; cubic micrometers, or femtoliters, fl); a measure of cell size. Used in classification of anemias to indicate if the RBC is normal size (**normocytic**), large (**macrocytic**), or small (**microcytic**). This will be explained further in the discussion of anemia, below.

- **RBC morphology** on peripheral smear – various diseases can cause changes in the shape and size of the RBC; these will be noted in the lab report. Their significance varies from disease to disease.

  Anisocytosis – variation in the size of RBCs (large, moderate, or small) as noted by the laboratory technician. Note that the red cell distribution width(see below) is the Coulter Counter's (automated CBC machine) equivalent to anisocytosis on the blood smear.

  Poikilocytosis – abnormally shaped RBCs

  Target cells – abnormal RBC characterized by a densely stained center surrounded by a pale, unstained ring circled by a dark, irregular bank; occur after splenectomy and in certain types of anemia (e.g., thalassemia).

- The **reticulocyte count** – not part of the routine CBC; reticulocytes are immature RBCs with a meshlike pattern of threads and particles at the site of the former nucleus; normally less than 1% of the circulating erythrocytes; elevated after hemorrhage or during recovery from anemia; the reticulocyte count needs to be corrected for anemia, yielding the **reticulocyte index**:

  Reticulocyte index = reticulocyte % X patient hct/normal hct

  The reticulocyte index is used to measure the appropriateness of the bone marrow response to anemia. In normal persons, as well as those with anemia and an appropriate bone marrow response, it should be close to 1. If lower, the BM response is inappropriate for the degree of anemia.

- The **erythrocyte sedimentation rate** (**ESR** or **sed rate**) measures the rate at which RBCs settle out of anticoagulated blood in one hour. It is **not** part of the routine CBC. The faster the settling, the higher the rate. Often called the **Westergren ESR**, normal in men is 0-15 mm/hr and in females, 0-20 mm/hr. The ESR is a nonspecific measurement of inflammation and should not be used as a screening test. It is most helpful for diagnosing and monitoring temporal arteritis, polymyalgia rheumatica, and artificial joint infections.

- The **red cell distribution width** (RDW) is a measurement of the amount that red blood cells vary in size. Normally, the red blood cells in a particular person's blood are similar in size. The normal RDW level is 10.2 to 14.5%. To determine what the possible cause of an abnormal RDW level is, a comparison is made to the mean corpuscular volume (MCV, defined above, a measure of cell size. Potential conditions in which variances in RDW and MCV are noted in the table below. [**Author's note**: I do not personally find the RDW terribly helpful in the initial diagnosis of anemia – see below].

MCV	RDW	POSSIBLE CAUSES:
Low	Normal	• Chronic disease • Thalassemia
Low	High	• Iron deficiency • Red blood cell fragmentation (artificial valve) • Thalassemia
Normal	Normal	• Abnormal hemoglobin • Any chronic disease (including chronic liver disease) • Hemorrhage • Hemolysis • Transfusion • Chronic lymphocytic leukemia • Hereditary spherocytosis
Normal	High	• Early iron or folate (or both) deficiency • Abnormal hemoglobin • Myelofibrosis
High	Normal	• Aplastic anemia • Preleukemia
High	High	• Folate of B-12 deficiency • Autoimmune hemolytic anemia • Cold agglutin disease (mycoplasma infection)

Note: Low RDW is usually due to either macrocytic anemia or microcytic anemia, where all the cells are either too large or too small (see below).

■ **Red Cell Disorders** – anemia and polycythemia

Anemia – anemia is defined as a lower than normal number of red blood cells.

1. Definition – since the RBC count is rarely used clinically, the most common way we define anemia is as low Hct and Hgb levels:

   • Hct < 42% (men), 37% (women)
   • Hgb < 14 g% (men), 12 g% (women)

15

2. Variables that affect hct determination – the factors below must always be kept in mind as they may lead to false-positive or false-negative diagnosis of anemia:

Variables that increase hct	Variables that decrease hct
Dehydration	Volume overload
Fingerstick (heelstick, earlobe) samples	Supine position
Prolonged tourniquet time	Capillary tube leak during centrifugation
Cold exposure	Automated techniques
Increased muscle activity	
Upright position	
Centrifugation tecnhiques	

3. General approach to anemia – the following illustrates the general thinking approach to a patient with anemia (low H/H):

- If the patient is anemic, are other cell lines involved? If so, then think of leukemia, acquired immunodeficiency, drug-induced bone marrow suppression or aplastic anemia

- Classify the anemia based on: (see below for how to use this information in a practical, clinically-relevant fashion)

    - **Cell size** [MCV or MCH] – normocytic, microcytic, macrocytic

    - **Intracellular hgb concentration** [MCHC] – normochromic, hypochromic, hyperchromic

    - **Mechanism** – decreased bone marrow production, bleeding, hemolysis

        - Anemia with an appropriate bone marrow response (reticulocytosis) suggests bleeding or hemolysis. Bleeding is far more common than is hemolysis.

        - Look at the rate of fall of the hct – with total marrow shutdown and no bleeding/hemolysis, hct falls no more than 3-4 hct points per week (1/120 of the RBC mass per day). If the fall is more rapid than this, in the absence of marked plasma volume changes, consider bleeding or hemolysis.

4. Practical clinical application of the approach to anemia – the "classical" approach to anemia has involved the above-named thinking process (cell size, intracellular hgb concentration, and mechanism). Practically speaking, there is an easier way that works *most* of the time and doesn't require a lot of details. I suggest that you try this approach first.

This method is based on determining the type of anemia based on the size of the red blood cell alone – this avoids the need to consider MCHC and mechanism – and both are sometimes confusing to non-hematologists. This method is based on the assumption that normal sized cells typically have normal hemoglobin and DNA within. Cells that have either abnormal hemoglobins or DNA tend to be either too big or too small. Metaphorically, I call cells that are either too big or too small, as measured by the MCV (too high or too low) to be "ugly." So, once identifying that anemia is present (i.e., H/H low), you should ask "are the cells ugly?" Really, what you are asking is whether or not the RBCs are normal sized. So, using the MCV, classify the anemia by cell sizes:

- Normal MCV (not "ugly") = normocytic anemia; the cells are normal sized; their DNA and hgb are normal. So these are normally functioning cells that are shaped normal. There just aren't enough of them (anemia).

- Low MCV ("ugly" = microcytic anemia; these cells are smaller than usual. Usually this indicates a hemoglobin problem.

- High MCV ("ugly") = macrocytic anemia; these cells are larger than usual. Usually this indicates a DNA problem.

The initial thinking is summarized in the figure below:

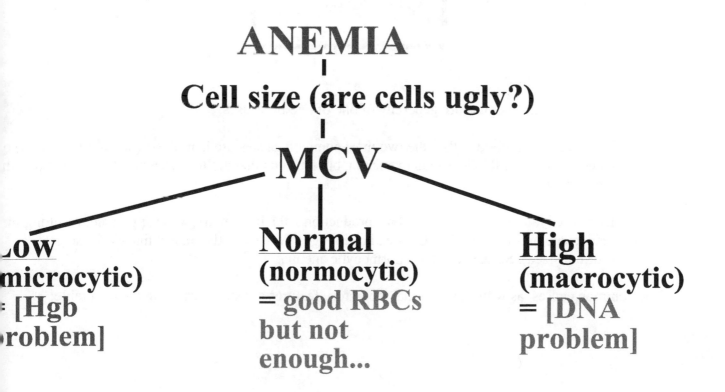

ANEMIA

Cell size (are cells ugly?)

MCV

**Low
(microcytic)
= [Hgb
problem]**

**Normal
(normocytic)
= good RBCs
but not
enough...**

**High
(macrocytic)
= [DNA
problem]**

Let's look in more detail at anemias with **normal MCV**, the **normocytic anemias**. Remember, the RBCs are normal, they're just aren't enough of them:

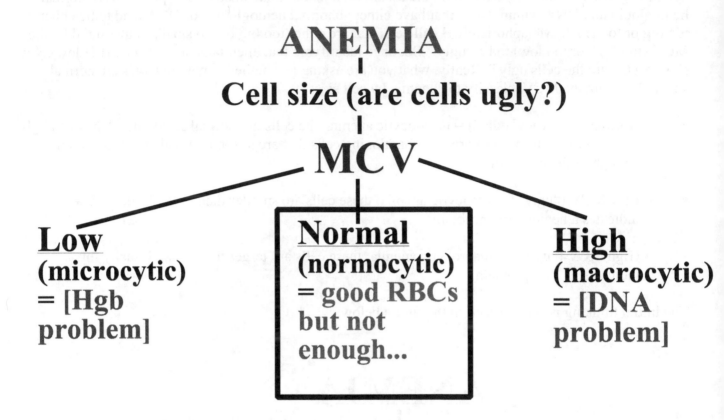

Causes of normocytic anemias are generally of one of two processes:

1.   Loss of normal blood cells – the two most common causes are hemolysis (hemolytic anemia) or bleeding. Loss of RBCs results in anemia, but the cells that are lost, as well as those that remain are normal.

2.   Decreased rate of bone marrow RBC production – the bone marrow is suppressed, resulting in inadequate production of RBCs (i.e., not enough). However, the ones it makes are normal (normal sized). So the result is a normocytic anemia.

The common causes, as well as additional laboratory features are summarized in the next table:

NORMOCYTIC ANEMIA (MCV NORMAL; NORMAL SIZED RBCS)

Cause	MCHC	Retic Index	Peripheral Smear	Comment
Hemolysis	WNL	appropriate for degree of anemia	often WNL; certain "funny looking cells" may suggest specific diagnoses (helmet cells = microangiopathic hemolysis)	MCV may be slightly inc if severe due to shift of early retics from bone marrow; think of with normochromic + normocytic anemia and no evidence of bleeding
Bleeding	WNL	appropriate for degree of anemia	usually WNL	H/H not reliable initially due to compensatory vasoconstriction and hemodilution; dec for several days after hemorrhage ceases; MCV may be slightly inc if severe due to shift of early retics from bone marrow
Renal failure	WNL	inappropriately low for degree of anemia	occasional spiculated ("burr") cells	dec production secondary to dec erythropoietin; mild thrombocytopenia common
Inflammatory or chronic disease (e.g., malignancy)	WNL	inappropriately low for degree of anemia	WNL	dec production + dec RBC survival; moderate anemia (hct not usu < 25%
Aplastic anemia	WNL	inappropriately low for degree of anemia	moderate anisocytosis	chemotherapy usually causes megaloblastic picture

Now, let's look at anemias with **low MCV**, the **microcytic anemias**. In this case, the hemoglobin is abnormal, causing the cell size to be decreased. The physical explanation for this is that abnormal hemoglobin proteins don't fold together properly – essentially the "cell scaffolding" is tighter-packed and the cells become smaller.

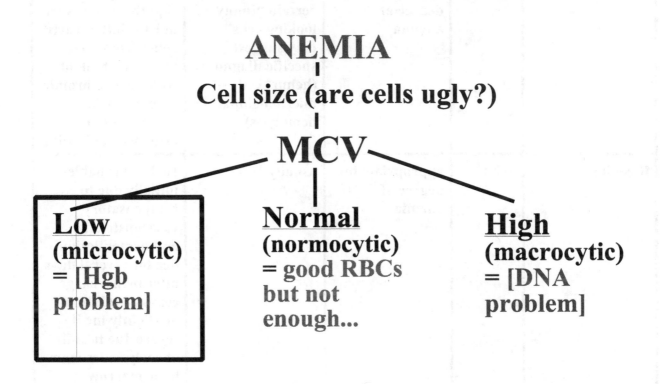

Common causes of microcytic anemias (due to impaired hemoglobin formation) are iron deficiency and thalassemia. These are summarized in the table below::

MICROCYTIC ANEMIA (LOW MCV, SMALL RBCS)

Cause	MCHC	Retic Index	Peripheral Smear	Comment
Iron deficiency	normal early; then low	low	poikilocytosis with small, hypochromic cells	either thrombocytosis or mild thrombocytopenia and leukopenia if severe
Thalassemia	normal to low	inc	microcytosis, target cells	anemia usually mild; common in Greeks and Italians

Finally, lets look at anemias with **high MCV**, the **macrocytic anemias**. In this case, the DNA is abnormal, causing the cell size to be increased. The physical explanation for this is that abnormal DNA doesn't pack together into the double helix configuration as readily as does normal DNA. This causes the cells to be larger. Common causes are summarized in the table below.

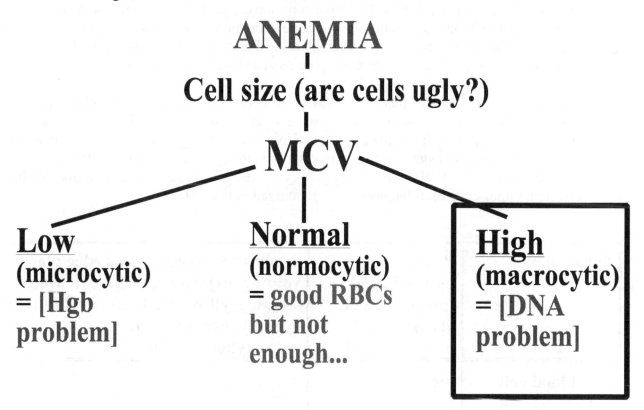

ANEMIA
Cell size (are cells ugly?)
MCV

Low (microcytic) = [Hgb problem]

Normal (normocytic) = good RBCs but not enough...

High (macrocytic) = [DNA problem]

MACROCYTIC ANEMIA (HIGH MCV, LARGE RBCS)

Cause	MCHC	Retic Index	Peripheral Smear	Comment
Liver disease	WNL	WNL	Target cells; no anisocytosis or poikilocytosis (A&P)	WBC/platelets variable; cells appear large due to lipid accumulation in RBC membrane
Megaloblastic anemia (folate or vitamin B12 deficiency [pernicious anemia]; severe alcoholism; drugs [DPH, methotrexate, TMP, 5-FU, 6-MP]))	WNL	low	marked A&P; teardrop-shaped cells; hypersegmented WBC nuclei	WBC/platelets often dec

Polycythemia is the opposite of anemia – an *increase* in the numbers of red cells, as manifested by elevated H/H. There are two types of polycythemia:

1. Primary polycythemia – this occurs in the absence of a secondary stimulus to increased bone marrow production of red cells. The most common cause is polycythemia vera, a tumor-like (though relatively benign) condition where the bone marrow gets out of control and produces excess numbers of normal red blood cells. Often abnormal numbers of white blood cells and platelets are also produced by the same process. The cause is uncertain.

2. Secondary polycythemia – this occurs due to some type of condition (see table below) that stimulates the bone marrow to produce excessive amounts of normal RBCs. The most common conditions have, in common, the presence of hypoxia (e.g., smoking, COPD). In an attempt to improve the body's oxygen carrying capacity, the kidneys produce more erythropoietin, leading to an increase in the H/H. In secondary polycythemia, platelets and WBCs are usually not affected. Other clinical differences are summarized in the table below:

Parameter	Primary polycythemia (polycythemia vera)	Secondary polycythemia (dec plasma volume, hypoxia, COPD, smoking, stress, erythropoietin producing tumors, cyanotic heart disease, carboxyhemoglobin)
Red blood cell mass	inc	inc
WBCs	usually inc	WNL
Platelets	usually inc	WNL
Platelet morphology	abnormal	WNL
Spleen size	usually inc	WNL
Itching	common	uncommon

■ White Cell Disorders

1. **Absolute counts** – occasionally, clinicians will want to determine the absolute numbers of one or more types of circulating WBC. This is called the absolute count and is calculated as follows:

Absolute count = total WBC count X differential % of individual cell types

The normal values for adults are as follows:

Neutrophils	1800-8000/ul
Eosinophils	0-600/ul
Basophils	0-200/ul
Lymphocytes	1000-5000/ul
Monocytes	0-1800/ul

2. **Too many cells** – **leukocytosis** usually only occurs due to elevation of **one** type of WBC and is given the name of the type of cell that shows the main increase; a proportional increase in leukocytes of all types is usually due to hemoconcentration. In certain diseases (e.g., measles, pertussis, and sepsis), the increase in the WBC is so great that the blood picture suggests leukemia (**leukemoid reaction**). In leukemia, though, the leukocytosis is permanent and progressive. Common causes of various types of leukocytosis are summarized in the table below.

Condition	Common causes
Neutrophilia	Acute and chronic inflammation Stress (emotional and physical) Infections Tumors Drugs (steroids, epinephrine, lithium) Splenectomy Hemorrhage Hemolytic anemia Seizures Myeloproliferative disorders
Eosinophilia	Parasitic infection Allergic reactions Dermatitis Hodgkins disease Myeloproliferative disease Adrenal insufficiency Chronic renal disease Radiotherapy Drugs Asthma Collagen vascular disease Hypereosinophilic syndromes
Basophilia	Hypersensitivity reactions Myeloproliferative disorders Postsplenectomy Inflammation
Monocytosis	Inflammation Malignancy Endocarditis Tuberculosis Collagen vascular disease Myeloproliferative syndromes Hodgkins disease Leukemias Neutropenia During recovery from agranulocytosis

Condition	Common causes
Neutrophilia	Acute and chronic inflammation Stress (emotional and physical) Infections Tumors Drugs (steroids, epinephrine, lithium) Splenectomy Hemorrhage Hemolytic anemia Seizures Myeloproliferative disorders
Lymphocytosis	Pertussis Chronic lymphocytic leukemia Thyrotoxicosis Infectious mononucleosis Cytomegalovirus infection Viral hepatitis Other viral illnesses Typhoid fever Allergic reactions Lymphosarcoma cell leukemia Acute lymphatic leukemia

3. **Too few cells** – the most common conditions resulting in too few WBCs are too few neutrophils (neutropenia) and too few lymphocytes (lymphopenia). Common causes of each are summarized in the tables below.

CAUSES OF NEUTROPENIA

Mechanism	Causes
Dec BM proliferation	Aplastic anemia (drug-induced; serious) Marrow infiltration (myelophthisis) Acute agranulocytosis (transient) Drug-induced (dose-related, idiosyncratic, hypersensitivity)
Ineffective BM production	Megaloblastic anemia (folate, vitamin B12 deficiency, drugs [methotrexate, hydroxyurea, DPH]) Preleukemia

Mechanism	Causes
Dec neutrophil survival	Leukocyte antibodies (uncommon)
Redistribution (margination)	Hypersplenism Overwhelming bacterial sepsis Viremia

CAUSES OF LYMPHOPENIA

Congenital immunodeficiency syndromes
Acquired immunodeficiency syndrome
Malignancy
Hodgkins disease
Chemotherapy
Radiotherapy
Collagen vascular disease
Inflammation
Corticosteroid excess
Uremia

■ **Platelet Disorders**

There are three common types of platelet disorders:

• Thrombocytopenia – too few platelets; the biggest risk here is bleeding. As long a the platelet count is > 50,000, clinically significant bleeding is unlikely to occur. When the count drops below 50,000, however, the risk increases progressively as the count goes lower.

• Disorders of platelet function – various conditions (especially drugs) can cause abnormal clotting function of platelets, *despite* normal platelet counts. So, the clinician must not just look at the platelet count, but the clinical picture as well.

• Thrombocytosis – too many platelets; the obvious risk is thrombosis. The risk of clinically significant clotting is greatest with platelet counts greater than one million, though elevations above 600,000 have also been noted to be problematic.

CAUSES OF THROMBOCYTOPENIA

Mechanism	Associated Diseases	Comments
Decreased survival, sequestration	Hypersplenism TTP Hemolytic uremic syndrome DIC Sepsis Immune thrombocytopenia (primary [ITP] or secondary [viruses, drugs, lupus])	If severe (< 10,000), consider immune process; large, elongated platelets on smear suggest destruction or sequestration (immature platelets released early); platelets normally survive for 10 days – 1/3 normally in spleen;
Decreased production	Myelophthisis Primary BM disorder Infection Drugs (thiazides, ETOH)	If severe (< 10,000), consider leukemia, aplastic anemia (including drugs); small platelets are old and suggest a production problem (e.g., aplastic anemia).
Ineffective production	Megaloblastic processes (folate, vitamin B12 deficiency; drugs)	Size varies; look for other evidence of megaloblastic development (inc MCV, hypersegmented WBC nuclei)

DISORDERS OF PLATELET FUNCTION

Type	Common conditions	Comment
Congenital	von Willebrand's disease Bernard-Soulier syndrome	Also Factor VIII deficiency with von Willebrand's
Acquired	Drugs (ASA, NSAIDs) Uremia Severe liver disease Multiple myeloma Leukemia	

CAUSES OF THROMBOCYTOSIS

Type	Common conditions	Comment
Myeloproliferative disorders	Polycythemia vera Primary thrombocythemia Agnogenic myeloid metaplasia Chronic granulocytic leukemia	Platelet counts typically > 1,000,000; morphology bizarre and function abnormal; bleeding common, especially when platelet count is very high; platelets may clump in microcirculation, causing thrombosis.
Secondary thrombocytosis	Inflammation Malignancy Hodgkins disease Acute bleeding Post-splenectomy Severe iron deficiency Chronic hypoxia (sleep apnea, COPD)	Does not cause a bleeding diathesis.

CHAPTER 3 – THE URINALYSIS
PARAMETERS MEASURED
THE TEST IN A "NUTSHELL"
NORMAL VALUES
PANIC VALUES
RESULTS IN A "NUTSHELL"
TEST DETAILS

CHAPTER 3 – THE URINALYSIS

The **UA** or **urinalysis** determines various parameters of the urine, including its' appearance under the microscope. Helps detect abnormalities where the kidneys are normal but excrete abnormal amounts o metabolic end products due to a specific disease; also helps detect and diagnose conditions of the kidneys or urinary tract.

- **Parameters measured:** Physical (color, appearance, specific gravity, pH), chemical (glucose, ketones, blood, protein, bilirubin, urobilinogen, nitrate, leukocyte esterase), and microscopic (casts, RBC, crystals, WBC epithelial cells)

- **The test in a "nutshell":** Measures the physical characteristics of the urine (SG, pH), the chemical characteristics using a chemically impregnated dipstick, and evaluates the urinary sediment under the microscope. Commonly ordered to evaluate dysuria, fluid balance, kidney status, liver function.

- **Normal values:**

PHYSICAL	CHEMICAL (DIPSTICK)	MICROSCOPIC
Color: pale yellow to amber Appearance: clear to slightly hazy Specific gravity: 1.015-1.025 pH: 4.5-8.0	Glucose: negative Ketones: negative Blood: negative Protein: negative Bilirubin: negative Urobilinogen: negative Nitrate for bacteria: negative Leucocyte esterase: negative	Casts: negative except for occasional hyaline RBC: rare or negative Crystals: negative WBC: negative or rare Epithelial cells: few

PANIC FINDINGS!!

Red urine negative for occult blood (porphyria)

Black or brown urine (blood)

Dip (+) for blood, microscopic (-) for RBC (myoglobinuria)

- **Results in a "nutshell":**

PARAMETER	IMPLICATIONS
Color	**Colorless** may indicate over hydration, nephritis, ETOH, diuretics, nervousness; **orange** may be due to concentrated urine, excess sweating, fever, small quantities of bile, Pyridium; **brownish yellow** or **greenish yellow** suggests bilirubin; **red** to **dark brown** suggests hemoglobin or myoglobin. Many drugs and foods alter urine color. See additional details under "color," below.
Appearance	**Cloudiness** may be due to RBC, WBC, or bacteria; many normal urines also appear cloudy.
Specific gravity	**Dec** with diabetes insipidus, glomerulonephritis, pyelonephritis, chronic renal failure; **inc** with diabetes mellitus, nephrosis, excessive water loss, SIADH; **fixed S.G.** (1.010) indicates severe renal damage.
pH	**Acidic** occurs in acidosis, uncontrolled diabetes, diarrhea, starvation, dehydration, CO_2 retention; **alkaline** occurs in UTI, salicylate intoxication, chronic renal failure, hyperventilation.
Glucose	**Inc** in endocrine disease (DM, thyrotoxicosis, Cushing's, acromegaly), brain injury, renal tubule disease, kidney inflammation; often **transiently elevated** in normal individuals after a heavy meal or during emotional stress. Poor screen/monitor for diabetes due to varying renal threshold for spilling glucose.
Ketones	**Positive** due to diabetes mellitus, starvation, fasting, high-fat diets, prolonged vomiting, anorexia, hyperthyroidism, fever, acute illness, alcoholism; in the nondiabetic indicates reduced carbohydrate metabolism and excessive fat metabolism.

Blood	**Positive** with free hemoglobin (**hemoglobinuria**), or myoglobin; **stippled** with RBCs (**hematuria**); **causes of hematuria** include infection, trauma, smoking, stones, cancer, exercise, glomerulonephritis; **causes of hemoglobinuria** include burn and crush injuries, transfusion reactions, malaria, hemolytic disorders, DIC, excessive exercise.
Protein	**Inc** with **kidney disease** (nephritis, glomerulonephritis, nephrosis, malignant hypertension, polycystic kidney disease, chronic urinary tract obstruction; **nonkidney disease** may also cause (e.g., fever, infection, trauma, leukemia, preeclampsia, diabetes, hypertension, lupus, poisonings). **Orthostatic proteinuria** is present in 15% of young, healthy adults.
Bilirubin	Any **trace** or **greater** of bilirubin in the urine is abnormal; **inc** levels occur in hepatitis and other liver diseases, obstructive biliary tract diseases (e.g., stones, tumors); **negative** in hemolytic disease.
Urobilinogen	**Inc** with RBC destruction (hemolysis, pernicious anemia), tissue hemorrhage, liver damage (biliary disease, cirrhosis, acute hepatitis), cholangitis; **Dec** or **absent** with biliary obstruction (stones, biliary inflammation, cancer of head of pancreas), suppression of gut flora (normally breakdown bilirubin to urobilinogen).
Nitrate for bacteria	**Positive** indicates significant bacteriuria; **negative** result does <u>not</u> rule out infection. Staph and strep UTIs are nitrate-negative.
Leucocyte esterase	**Positive** suggests presence of leukocytes in the urine and UTI; **negative** suggests absence of leukocytes, but does not definitively r/o UTI; vaginal discharge or bleeding can cause false positive.
Casts	**Presence** of any type of cast other than an occasional hyaline cast indicates severe renal disease (e.g., nephrotic syndrome, glomerulonephritis, pyelonephritis, kidney failure). **RBC casts** always indicate hemorrhage usually due to glomerulonephritis, renal infarction, collagen vascular disease, or SBE; **WBC casts** indicate infection of the renal parenchyma (pyelonephritis, acute glomerulonephritis); **epithelial casts** suggest nephrosis, heavy metal poisoning, acute tubular necrosis, glomerulonephritis.

Cells (RBC, WBC, epithelial cells)	**RBCs** (> 2/HPF [high power field]) compatible with kidney trauma, pyelonephritis, SLE, kidney stones, cystitis, prostatitis, GU malignancy, hemophilia, malignant hypertension; rule out presence of menstrual blood, vaginal bleeding, or perineal trauma in the female patient. **WBCs [leukocytes]** (>50/HPF) usually indicate bacterial infection in the urinary tract; in smaller numbers may be due to renal disease, urinary tract disease, fever, exercise, appendicitis, bladder tumors. A **few squamous cells** are normal.
Crystals	Depends on type and number of crystals; may be **normal** (amorphous urates, few uric acid, small calcium oxalate, calcium carbonate, calcium phosphate, amorphous phosphates); **inc** due to gout (uric acid), severe liver disease (bilirubin), chronic renal disease (calcium oxalate).
Bacteria	Normally the urine is sterile; the presence of bacteria indicates UTI

■ **Test details**

1. **Physical properties**

   ▸ **Color** – darker amber color may be related to inc SG; many drugs and foods cause changes in the urine color.

Color	Potential Causes
Red	beets, cascara and senna laxatives (alkaline urine)
Brown	rhubarb
Reddish brown	cascara and senna laxatives (acid urine)
Orange	Pyridium (phenazopyridine); oral anticoagulants
Rust-yellow	sulfonamides
Pink to red	DPH, diocytl calcium sulfosuccinate (Doxidan), phenolphthalein (Ex-Lax)
Purple-red	phenolphthalein (Ex-Lax)
Bright yellow	Riboflavin
Blue/green	methylene blue, vitamin B complex, amitriptyline
Pale blue	triamterene (Dyrenium, Diazide)
Brown-black	iron

▸ **Appearance** – generally, one of the first observations made on the urine. pH changes may cause proteins to precipitate, resulting in cloudy urine; this is often of no pathological significance; UTI can also cause turbidity as well as semen or vaginal discharges mixed with urine. Normal urine turns cloudy following refrigeration due to precipitation of proteins.

▸ **Specific gravity** – measures kidney's ability to concentrate and dilute the urine; compares the weight of urine against the weight of distilled water, which has SG of 1.000; normally varies inversely with the amount of urine excreted. If the SG becomes **fixed** at 1.010 (**isosthenuria**), the kidney has lost its ability to both concentrate and to dilute the urine. Isosthenuria is an indication of <u>severe</u> renal damage. A patient who ha recently received radiopaque XR contrast media may have falsely elevated readings; large quantities of proteinuria may have the same effect.

▸ **pH** – indicates the kidneys' ability to maintain normal hydrogen ion concentrations in the plasma and extracellular fluid; reabsorb sodium and secrete hydrogen and ammoniu to maintain pH. Urine pH varies based on diet – a high animal protein diet produces acidic urine; a diet high in fruits and vegetables produces an alkaline urine. Certain types of kidney stones are more prone to occur in specific acid-base environments: **acidic** (uric acid, calcium oxalate, cystine), **alkaline** (calcium phosphate, calcium carbonate, magnesium phosphate).

2. **Chemical properties (dipstick)**

▸ **Glucose** – glucose is present in the glomerular filtrate, but it reabsorbed by the proxima tubule. If the blood glucose level exceeds the reabsorption capacity (**renal threshold**) o the tubules, glucose will spill into the urine. **Glucosuria** is not always an indication of diabetes – stress or a heavy meal can result in transient spillage as well. A fasting bloo sugar determination is far more helpful than urine testing in determining the diagnosis o diabetes mellitus. Similarly, fingerstick blood sugar determinations are far more accurate than urine tests for on-going monitoring of diabetic patients.

▸ **Ketones** – result from the metabolism of fatty acid and fat. There are two main ketones beta-hydroxybutyric acid (BOHB), and acetoacetate – they interconvert, depending on the pH. Most dipsticks and Acetest tablets only detect acetoacetate. If a patient is acidotic (e.g., diabetic ketoacidosis), BOHB predominates. As the pH normalizes durin treatment, the equilibrium of the reaction shifts so that BOHB interconverts to acetoacetate. This is called the **redox shift**. Thus, transiently, there appears to be an **increase** rather than the expected **decrease** in ketones. Actually, what is happening is that the <u>proportion</u> of BOHB is <u>decreasing</u> and that of acetoacetate is <u>increasing</u>. Since the test only measures acetoacetate, it appears that the ketones have gone up. As the process continues to correct, and <u>all</u> the ketones are cleared from the body, the total amounts of **both** BOHB and acetoacetate will decrease, resulting in a decreased reading

▸ **Blood** – free hemoglobin in the urine is **hemoglobinuria** and, by itself, is usually related to conditions outside the urinary tract (e.g., hemolysis). Intact RBCs in the urine, or **hematuria**, indicates bleeding somewhere in the urinary tract. Usually, hemoglobinuria accompanies hematuria, so microscopic examination of the urine is necessary to differentiate the two conditions. If the urine is dipstick positive for occult blood but no RBC are seen on microscopic examination, suspect **myoglobinuria**, since hemoglobin cross-reacts with myoglobin on the dipstick test.

▸ **Protein** – the glomerular membranes normally prevent passage of protein from the blood to the filtrate; the presence of protein in the urine is a strong indication of kidney disease; often a 24-hour urine collection is then required to determine the degree of **proteinuria** over an extended period of time.

The Kinetics of Bilirubin

RETICULOENDOTHELIAL SYSTEM

RBCs are broken down in the RE system (particularly the spleen) releasing hemoglobin; globin is removed, leaving heme. Heme is metabolized in the RE system first to biliverdin, then to bilirubin. At this stage, the bilirubin is non-water soluble or **unconjugated** (**indirect**). The RE system then releases the unconjugated bilirubin into the plasma.

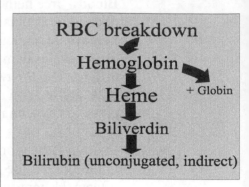

RBC breakdown

Hemoglobin

Heme + Globin

Biliverdin

Bilirubin (unconjugated, indirect)

PLASMA

Unconjugated bilirubin binds avidly with albumin in the plasma. This complex does **not** appear in urine, but is present in other body fluids (e.g., CSF, joint effusions, cysts) in direct proportion to the albumin content of the fluid. It is absent from true secretions (e.g., tears, saliva, and pancreatic juice). The unconjugated bilirubin-albumin complex is transported in the plasma to the liver, where it is taken up into the hepatocyte.

Unconjugated Bilirubin + Albumin

BU-A complex in plasma

Liver   Body Fluids

LIVER

Once the complex enters the hepatic cell, the albumin dissociates from unconjugated bilirubin. Unconjugated bilirubin is not water soluble, and needs to be converted to a water soluble form in order to be excreted from the liver to the bile. The conjugation process converts bilirubin primarily to bilirubin glucuronide (BRG). This reaction takes place in the endoplasmic reticulum of the hepatocytes. The **conjugated bilirubin** (or BRG, **direct bilirubin**) is then secreted into the bile.

BU-A Complex

Non-water soluble BU + A

Conjugation

[BRG] Water-soluble

Bilirubin glucuronide (conjugated, d

Bile

GALL BLADDER

BRG enters the gall bladder via the **hepatic duct** and becomes part of the bile. During the digestive process, bile (including BRG) is secreted into the intestine.

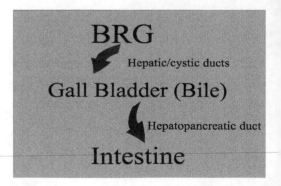

BRG

Hepatic/cystic ducts

Gall Bladder (Bile)

Hepatopancreatic duct

Intestine

INTESTINE

Here, some of the BRG is excreted in the stool. The remainder is metabolized by lower intestinal and colonic bacteria into urobilinogen (UB). UB may be excreted in the stool or reabsorbed via the portal circulation to the liver.

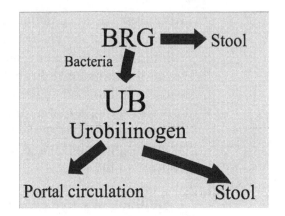

PORTAL SYSTEM

UB that is not excreted in the stool returns, via the hepatoportal system, to the liver.

LIVER

Here, some UB is re-excreted into the bile, then into the intestine. The rest is transported via the blood stream to the kidney.

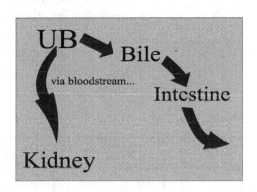

KIDNEY

UB from the liver is filtered and excreted by the kidneys. Normally, only a small amount is excreted, but there is always some. Normal urinary UB = 0 - trace.

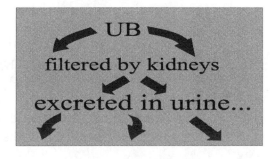

- **Bilirubin** – formed in the spleen and bone marrow as a breakdown product of hemoglobin; it is transported to the liver, where it is conjugated (made water soluble), secreted in bile, and excreted in the stool. Any process that increases the level of conjugated bilirubin leads to a positive test. Normally, there is no detectable bilirubin in the urine, despite the presence of a small amount of urobilinogen. Bilirubin often appears in the urine before other signs of liver disease are noted (jaundice, weakness). Unconjugated bilirubin is tightly bound to albumin, thus not filtered by the renal glomeruli. Only conjugated bilirubin appears in the urine.

- **Urobilinogen** – formed in the intestine by bacterial action on bilirubin; some is excreted in the stool, while the rest travels to the liver via the portal circulation. Most is metabolized in the liver and excreted in the bile; traces that are not metabolized by the liver are carried to the kidneys and excreted in the urine.

  - Urobilinogen is colorless and is **increased** by any condition that causes an increase in bilirubin production (e.g., hemolytic anemia) and/or prevents the liver from normally removing the reabsorbed urobilinogen from the portal circulation (e.g., hepatocellular disease).

  - **Decreased** urinary levels result when normal amounts of bilirubin are not excreted into the GI tract (and then broken down to UB in the intestine and colon), indicating a partial or complete obstruction of the bile ducts (e.g., cholelithiasis, cholangitis, pancreatic cancer) or in severe liver disease where the liver cannot properly absorb it, or if the intestinal flora are suppressed and unable to make it from conjugated bilirubin..

Test	Normal	Hemolysis	Liver Disease	Biliary Obstruction
Urine urobilinogen	WNL	Increased	Increased	Low or absent
Urine bilirubin	Negative	Negative	Positive or negative	Positive

- **Nitrate** – an indirect indication of bacteriuria; helpful especially if UTI is asymptomatic (e.g., pregnancy, diabetes, elderly, young children). Any shade of pink(on the urinary dipstick) indicates the presence of nitrate-producing organisms and significant bacteriuria. Since certain organisms don't form nitrate (e.g., staph and strep), a negative test does <u>not</u> rule out UTI. Vitamin C (ascorbic acid) can produce false negative results.

➤ **Leukocyte esterase** – esterase is released by WBCs in the urine; the intensity of the purple color on the dipstick is proportional to the concentration of WBC in the sample; detects both intact and lysed leukocytes, as well as WBC casts. A urine sample positive for both nitrate and leukocyte esterase is <u>strong</u> evidence favoring UTI.

Microscopic properties

➤ **Casts** – often indicate tubular or glomerular disorders; the width of the cast indicates the diameter of the tubule responsible for its formation.

- **Broad (waxy) casts** (five RBC in width) form in the collecting tubule and are composed of homogenous, yellowish material; often called **renal failure casts**, they indicate severe kidney dysfunction.

- **RBC casts** are always abnormal and usually indicate hemorrhage or severe inflammation (e.g., glomerulonephritis)

- **WBC casts** indicate dysfunction of the renal parenchyma and are most common in pyelonephritis. They may also occur in acute glomerulonephritis or interstitial inflammation of the kidney.

- **Epithelial casts** are common when the tubule epithelium has been damaged (e.g., nephrosis, amyloidosis, heavy metal poisoning, glomerulonephritis, acute tubular necrosis).

- **Hyaline casts** are clear, colorless casts formed when the Tamm-Horsfall protein (the main constituent of urinary protein) precipitates and gels in the kidneys; a few may be WNL; many indicate nephrotic syndrome (along with significant proteinuria), chronic renal disease, diabetic nephropathy, nephritis, or malignant hypertension; stress may also cause the temporary presence of hyaline casts.

- **Granular casts** are homogenous, coarsely granular, colorless, and very dense. They are abnormal and often found in acute tubular necrosis, advanced glomerulonephritis, pyelonephritis, and chronic lead poisoning.

Casts – Cellular and acellular...

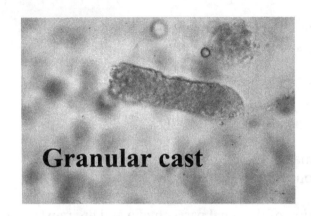

Granular cast

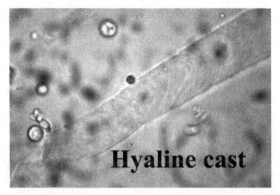

Hyaline cast

Acellular casts = RENAL FAILURE

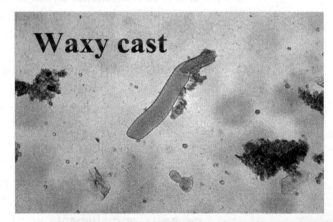

Waxy cast

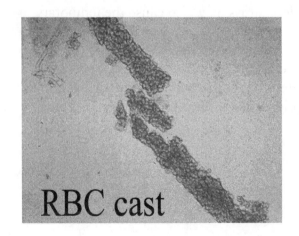

RBC cast

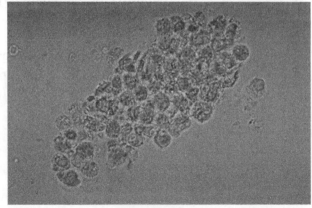

WBC Cast

Cellular casts = PYELONEPHRITIS

- **Cells (RBCs, WBCs, epithelial cells)** – though a few **RBCs** may occasionally appear in the urine, generally these come from the kidney and may indicate serious renal disease. **WBCs** may originate from anywhere in the genitourinary tract; > 50 cells per high powered field generally indicates acute infection. An occasional **renal epithelial cell** is not unusual, but large numbers are abnormal (e.g., acute tubular damage, acute glomerulonephritis, salicylate overdose).

- **Crystals** – these may be identified by their specific appearance and solubility characteristics; they may be asymptomatic or may be associated with stone formation.
- **Bacteria** – no bacteria should be present in the urine; sometimes a gram stain of the urine sediment is helpful in making a diagnosis.

CHAPTER 4 – CHEMISTRY PROFILES
PARAMETERS MEASURED
THE TEST IN A "NUTSHELL"
NORMAL VALUES
PANIC VALUES
RESULTS IN A "NUTSHELL"
TEST DETAILS
  SODIUM
  POTASSIUM
  CHLORIDE
  CALCIUM
  PHOSPHORUS
  MAGNESIUM
  BLOOD SUGAR (GLUCOSE)
  BUN (BLOOD UREA NITROGEN)
  CREATININE
  URIC ACID

CHAPTER 4 – CHEMISTRY PROFILES

- **Parameters measured:** Any one of a number of measurements of the serum concentration of a given compound; often part of an automated examination (e.g., SMA 6, 12, 20) that determines several specific parameters from a single sample of serum.

- **The test in a "nutshell":** Exactly what each "panel" covers is determined by the particular machine or laboratory used. Normals may vary widely between labs and/or machines. Typical tests include:

  ▸ **Electrolytes** (Na, K, Cl, HCO_3, Ca, Mg) – the basic "building block" chemicals of the body; alterations in the electrolytes can result in, as well as be the result of, numerous disease processes.

  ▸ **Blood sugar** – important to measure in the diagnosis of diabetes, as well as in altered levels of consciousness. Low blood sugar (hypoglycemia) may result in unusual neurological or behavioral abnormalities.

  ▸ **Kidney function** (BUN, Cr) – measure the excretory function of the kidney.

  ▸ **Uric acid** – elevated in gout. Commonly measured on multipanel tests.

- **Normal values:**

Test	Normal value (adult)
Sodium (Na^+)	135-145 mEq/L
Potassium (K^+)	3.5-5.3 mEq/L
Chloride (Cl^-)	98-106 mmol/L or mEq/L
Bicarbonate (HCO_3^-)	23-30 mmol/L
Calcium (Ca^{2+})	8.6-10.0 mg/dl
Magnesium (Mg^{2+})	1.3-2.1 mEq/L
Blood sugar (BS)	65-110 mg/dl
Blood urea nitrogen (BUN)	7-18 mg/dl

Creatinine (Cr)	0.6-1.3 mg/dl
Uric acid	Men: 3.5-7.2 mg/dl; women: 2.6-6.0 mg/dl

PANIC VALUES!!

BS < 40 mg/dl or > 450 mg/dl
BUN > 100 mg/dl
Ca^{2+} (total) < 6 mg/dl (tetany and convulsions)
Ca^{2+} (total) > 13 mg/dl (cardiotoxicity, arrhythmias, coma)
Cl^- < 70 or > 120 mEq/L (mmol/L)
Cr > 10 mg/dl (nondialysis patients)
HCO_3^- < 6.0 mmol/L (significant acidosis)
K^+ < 2.5 mEq/L or > 7.0 mEq/L (arrhythmias)
Mg^{2+} < 1.0 mEq/L (tetany)
Mg^{2+} > 15 mEq/L (respiratory paralysis, cardiac arrest)
Na^+ < 120 mEq/L (weakness, neurologic symptoms)
Na^+ > 155 mEq/L (cardiovascular collapse)

- **Results in a "nutshell":**

PARAMETER	IMPLICATIONS
Sodium (Na^+)	Reflects changes in water and salt balance; urinary sodium levels may be more helpful for altered Na^+ balance. Low levels usually reflect a relative excess of body water.
Potassium (K^+)	Evaluates changes in body potassium levels; these may change quickly, depending upon pH and hydration status. Changes, either too high or too low, can rapidly lead to dangerous cardiac dysrhythmias.
Chloride (Cl^-)	Alterations of chloride alone are rarely a primary problem; very important in correction of hypokalemic alkalosis; potassium supplementation alone will not correct without chloride as well.

Bicarbonate (HCO_3^-)	Reflects the CO_2 content of the blood, 95% of which is bicarbonate (HCO_3^-); may also be called **carbon dioxide content**. Alterations reflect changes in the acid-base balance of the blood. A general measure of the alkalinity or acidity present.
Calcium (Ca^{2+})	Measures the concentration of total calcium in the blood; reflects parathyroid function (elevated in hyperparathyroidism), calcium metabolism (decreased in vitamin D deficiency), and malignant disease (hypercalcemia is a common paraneoplastic syndrome).
Magnesium (Mg^{2+})	An index of metabolic activity as well as an evaluation of renal function and electrolyte status; levels either too high or too low can result in life-threatening problems.
Blood sugar (BS)	Diagnostic accuracy for diabetes depends upon whether or not obtained in fasting state; random tests (e.g., fingerstick) helpful to monitor diabetes or in suspected hypoglycemia.
Blood urea nitrogen (BUN)	Serves as a gross index of glomerular function as well as the production and excretion of urea; influenced by tissue necrosis, protein catabolism (GI bleeding), and the rate at which the kidneys excrete urea nitrogen.
Creatinine (Cr)	A very specific and sensitive test for kidney disease; in chronic renal failure, though, BUN level correlates better with uremic symptoms than Cr.
Uric acid	Elevation occurs with excessive cell breakdown and catabolism of nucleic acids (gout), excessive production and destruction of cells (leukemia), or inability to excrete (renal failure).

- **Test details**

Sodium (Na^+)

> ▸ Na^+ is the most abundant ECF cation.

> ▸ **Functions**: maintain osmotic pressure, acid-base balance, transmit nerve impulses

> ▸ **Control of Na^+ level** – four types of stimuli affect primarily the kidney, which then leads to changes in the $[Na^+]$:

Increased BP in the right atrium → release of *atrial natriuretic hormone* (ANH)	Increased osmolality affects hypothalamic neurons; decreased BP affects baroreceptors in the aortic arch, carotid sinuses, and atrium. Both of these stimuli → release of *anti-diuretic hormone* (ADH) from the posterior pituitary	Low BP stimulates *renin* secretion from the kidney; renin stimulates production of *angiotensin II*, which then stimulates formation of *aldosterone* by the adrenal cortex	Increased [K^+] levels in the blood stimulate *aldosterone* secretion by the adrenal cortex

THE KIDNEYS ARE AFFECTED BY THE ABOVE, LEADING TO THE CHANGES BELOW

ANH increases Na^+ excretion and water loss via urine, leading to a decrease in the BP	*ADH* increases water absorption, which decreases osmolality and increases BP	*Aldosterone* stimulates sodium ion and water reabsorption (K^+ excretion) in the kidney, leading to increased BP	*Aldosterone* increases the rate of potassium secretion in the kidneys, leading to lower [K^+]

- ▸ **Decreased** Na^+ occurs in severe burns, CHF, excessive fluid loss, excess IV fluids, Addison's disease (lack of adrenal steroids impairs sodium reabsorption), nephritis, malabsorption, DKA, diuretics, edema (dilutional), large amounts of water by mouth, hypothyroidism.

- ▸ **Increased** Na^+ occurs in dehydration, insufficient water intake, primary aldosteronism, coma, Cushing's disease, diabetes insipidus.

► **Clinical correlation**:

Problem	Subjective	Objective	Emergency Rx
Hyponatremia	Lethargy, confusion, seizures, coma	Edema, altered LOC, venous distension, tachycardia, hypotension, tachycardia, decreased urine output; weight gain	In acute hyponatremia, rapidly correct to 120-125 mEq/L. Fluid restriction if volume-expanded; if hypovolemic, isotonic NaCl; occasionally loop diuretics (furosemide) + fluids if markedly volume expanded; no role for hypertonic saline
Hypernatremia	Thirst, restlessness, seizures	Fever, dry mucous membranes, acute pulmonary edema, edema, weight gain	Fluids, ADH replacement in SIADH

Correct sodium abnormalities over the period of time you think they took to evolve. Acute hyper- or hyponatremia may be treated fairly rapidly, as outlined above. In both chronic hypernatremia and hyponatremia, the brain has already corrected for the osmolar changes (new "set point"). Changing the [Na$^+$] rapidly, either way, could lead to significant neurologic deterioration. In chronic hyponatremia, raise the [Na$^+$] no faster than 0.5 mEq/L/hr until it reaches 120 mEq/L. In chronic hypernatremia, lower the [Na$^+$] no faster than 1 mEq/L every 2 hours.

Potassium (K$^+$)

► The major intracellular cation; 90% within the cell; damaged tissue releases K$^+$ into the blood. The ratio of ECF to ICF K$^+$ establishes the resting membrane potential of cells. Factors that regulate the distribution of K$^+$ between the ECF and the ICF:

- Insulin – promotes cellular uptake.

- Aldosterone – affects the tissue distribution and regulates renal excretion; higher levels lead to increased excretion via the kidneys. Aldosterone secretion from the adrenal cortex is stimulated by elevated [K$^+$] and by angiotensin II (see above regarding sodium)

- Catecholamines (e.g., epinephrine) – cause movement of K$^+$ into cells; mediated by beta-adrenergic receptors (blocked by beta-blockers).

- Acid-base balance – acidosis increases serum [K$^+$]; alkalosis decreases

47

- 80-90% of K^+ excreted into the urine; the kidneys don't conserve K^+ – 40 to 50 mEq are still excreted daily even without any intake (obligatory urinary loss) – thus, inadequate ingestion may result in a serious deficiency without any other concomitant disease process.

- **Major functions**:

  - Nerve conduction
  - Muscle function
  - Acid-base balance
  - Osmotic pressure
  - Rate and force of heart contraction

- **Decreased** with shifting K^+ into cells (alkalosis, excess glucose such as during a GTT), K^+ loss from GI and biliary tracts (diarrhea, vomiting, excessive sweating, malabsorption), increased renal excretion (primary aldosteronism, excessive licorice ingestion, diuretics), and reduced K^+ intake (starvation).

  GI loss is the most frequent cause of K^+ deficiency; IV fluid administration without adequate K^+ supplementation is the most frequent cause of K^+ depletion.

- **Increased** with shifting K^+ out of cells (acidosis, decreased insulin, cell damage as in burns, accidents, DIC), inadequate renal excretion (renal failure, other kidney disease, Addison's disease, aldosterone deficiency [normally causes retention of Na^+ and renal excretion of K^+]), and excessive K^+ intake (potassium penicillin). Also, hemolysis of drawn blood will artificially and significantly elevate K^+ reading – opening and closing the fist ten times with a tourniquet in place → 10-20% inc in $[K^+]$.

Problem	Subjective	Objective	Emergency Rx
Hyperkalemia	Restlessness, cramping, diarrhea; muscle weakness, paralysis	EKG changes (peaked T waves, flattening of P waves and widening of QRS, disappearance of P waves, sine wave QRS, VT, VF)	Ca^{2+} to antagonize cardiac membrane effects; insulin + glucose + bicarbonate to shift K^+ into cells, ion exchange resins and diuretics to eliminate from the body; dialysis as last resort
Hypokalemia	Thirst, muscular irritability, lethargy	EKG changes (flattening of T waves, appearance of U waves, ectopy)	Depends on K^+ shifts (may just need to correct pH); no greater than 20 mEq/hr IV without EKG monitoring

Chloride (Cl⁻)

- Primarily in extracellular space as sodium chloride or hydrochloric acid.

- Maintains cellular integrity via influence on osmotic pressure, acid-base, and water balance.

- Increases or decreases in response to other ion concentrations; if bicarbonate drops in metabolic acidosis, there is a reciprocal rise in [Cl⁻]; if aldosterone causes an increase in the reabsorption of Na^+, there is also an indirect increase in chloride absorption.

- Excreted with cations during massive diuresis from any cause.

- Lost from GI tract when vomiting, diarrhea, or intestinal fistulas occur. [Cl⁻] is relatively high in gastric juices; prolonged vomiting may → considerable chloride loss.

- The least important electrolyte to measure in an emergency.

- Must give chloride along with potassium in hypokalemic alkalosis.

- Remains at near normal levels in the presence of severe renal failure.

- **Increased** in dehydration, Cushing's syndrome, hyperventilation (respiratory alkalosis), metabolic disorders, hyperparathyroidism, renal tubular acidosis, diabetes insipidus.
- **Decreased** in severe vomiting, chronic respiratory acidosis, massive gastric suction, burns, metabolic alkalosis, diabetes, Addison's disease, salt-losing diseases, overhydration.

Bicarbonate (HCO_3^-) [sometimes called total CO_2 content]

- More than 95% of plasma total CO_2 content is contributed by HCO_3^- (bicarbonate) which is regulated by the kidneys; this parameter gives virtually no indication of lung function since dissolved CO_2 gas (regulated by the lungs) constitutes only 5% of the total CO_2 in the blood.

- **Increased** in severe vomiting (loss of HCl from the stomach), emphysema (chronic compensation for respiratory acidosis), hyperaldosteronism

- **Decreased** in severe diarrhea (loss of alkali from colon), starvation, acute renal failure, salicylate toxicity, diabetic ketoacidosis, metabolic acidosis of nearly any kind.

▸ **Tidbits on metabolic acidoses**

- **Serum ketone level** – elevated in diabetic ketoacidosis; also in alcoholic ketoacidosis. Make certain to measure *serum* ketones, not urine ketones. Urine levels go up with mild dehydration, in the absence of ketoacidosis. To confirm a true ketoacidosis, elevated serum ketone levels are required.

- **Lactate levels** – values over 2 mmol/L poor prognostic sign; can be monitored by bedside device. Even in patients with liver disease, who are said to generate increased levels, elevated levels above 2.2 mM were still noted to correlate with tissue hypoxia, clinical evidence of shock, and with increased hospital mortality (Am J Med 83, July 1987, 77-82).

- **The anion-gap** – reflects concentrations of unmeasured anions that are present in the ECF (e.g., phosphates, sulfates, ketone bodies, lactate, and proteins) to maintain electrical neutrality. Their levels increase in certain types of metabolic acidoses.

  $AG = Na^+ - (Cl^- + HCO_3^-)$ and the normal value is < 12 mEq/L. An alternative formula incorporates the K^+ value: $AG = (Na^+ + K^+) - (Cl^- + HCO_3^-)$; here the normal value is < 16 mEq/L. Either formula is acceptable.

If a metabolic acidosis is present, calculate the anion gap – if it is increased ("widened"), then the patient has a **wide-anion gap metabolic acidosis** due to the production of excess metabolic acids. Possible causes include (the acronym spells "SLUMPED"):

S --	Salicylate intoxication
L --	Lactic acidosis
U --	Uremia (renal failure), underfed (fasting, starvation)
M --	Methanol ingestion
P --	Paraldehyde OD (rare)
E --	Ethanol (alcoholic ketoacidosis), ethylene glycol ingestion
D --	Diabetic ketoacidosis

If the anion gap is normal, the patient has a **non-anion gap metabolic acidosis**, and the above causes can usually be excluded. In this case, common causes include hyperchloremic acidoses and renal tubular acidosis.

Calcium (Ca^{2+})

▸ 98-99% of body Ca^{2+} is stored in the skeleton and teeth

▸ 50% of serum Ca^{2+} is protein-bound, the rest is ionized; only ionized form can be used in muscular contraction, cardiac function, transmission of nerve impulses

▸ Since 50% is protein bound, a decrease in serum albumin will result in a profound decrease in total serum calcium – consider obtaining **ionized calcium levels** (requires special test and preparation of blood).

▸ Calcium levels are influenced by many factors-- parathyroid hormone, calcitonin, vitamin D, estrogens, androgens, carbohydrates, and lactose.

- Decreased blood calcium → **parathyroid hormone** secretion from parathyroid glands.

- Parathyroid hormone increases Ca^{2+} reabsorption in kidney, resorption from bone, and increases **vitamin D** synthesis by the kidney (increases GI Ca^{2+} absorption).

- **Calcitonin**, secreted by the thyroid gland in response to increased blood calcium levels, decreases calcium resorption from bone, leading to a lower serum level.

► **Functions of calcium** in the body include bone and teeth formation, blood clotting, muscle contraction, nerve impulse conduction (especially in the heart). **Hypercalcemia** decreases the permeability of the cell membrane to sodium ions, preventing normal depolarization of nerve and muscle cells. **Hypocalcemia** increases the permeability of cell membranes to sodium ions, causing spontaneous action potential generation.

► Causes of **hypercalcemia** include hyperparathyroidism (parathyroid adenoma, hyperplasia of the parathyroid glands, hypophosphatemia), cancer (metastatic bone cancers, lung, breast, thyroid, kidney, liver, and pancreas, Hodgkins disease, multiple myeloma), granulomatous disease, hyperthyroidism, Paget's disease of bone, prolonged immobilization, excessive intake of vitamin D, milk-alkali syndrome (excessive intake of milk and antacids), drugs (thiazide diuretics impair urinary calcium excretion), magnesium deficiency (malabsorption; corrects with Mg^{2+} supplementation alone most of the time).

> *Hyperparathyroidism and cancer are the most common causes of hypercalcemia..*

► Causes of **hypocalcemia** include pseudohypocalcemia (reflection of decreased albumin levels), hypoparathyroidism (primary rare, surgical removal of parathyroid glands, GI disorders, renal calcium wasting), hyperphosphatemia (renal failure, laxative intake, cytotoxic drugs), malabsorption (sprue, celiac disease, pancreatic dysfunction), severe acute pancreatitis, alkalosis (calcium ions bind to protein – common in hyperventilation, renal failure, alcoholism, cirrhosis.

> *Low serum albumin is the most common cause of decreased total calcium.*

▸ **Clinical correlations**

Problem	Subjective	Objective	Emergency Rx
Hypercalcemia	Lethargy, drowsiness, depression, impaired ability to concentrate, confusion, coma; muscle weakness, nausea, vomiting, anorexia, constipation, abdominal pain, joint pains; ["Abdominal **moans**, joint **groans**, and fatigue **overtones**"]; polyuria, polydipsia, kidney stones	Proximal muscle weakness, hyporeflexia; hypertension, shortened QT interval, bradycardia, increased sensitivity to digitalis	Reverse underlying process; IV saline, furosemide (avoid thiazides), glucocorticoids, calcitonin (inhibits osteoclastic bone resorption and increases urinary calcium excretion); mithramycin (decreases osteoclastic activity); dialysis
Hypocalcemia	Paresthesias (circumoral, fingers, and toes), carpal pedal spasm, laryngospasm, bronchospasm, blepharospasm, tetany, seizures, papilledema, CHF	(+) Chvostek's sign (abnormal spasm of facial muscles elicited by light taps on the facial nerve); (+) Trousseau's sign (BP cuff inflated > systolic BP for 3 minutes → carpal spasm); prolonged QT interval (torsades de pointes), heart block	IV calcium gluconate, 1 amp over 5-10 minutes; correct concomitant hypomagnesemia.

Magnesium (Mg^{2+})

▸ Concentrated in bone, cartilage, and within the cell.

▸ Required for use of ATP as a source of energy.

- **Major functions**:

  - Cofactor in many enzyme systems (carbohydrate metabolism, protein synthesis, nucleic acid synthesis, muscular contraction)
  - Regulates neuromuscular irritability (along with sodium and calcium)
  - Regulation of blood clotting

- Intimately tied together with calcium; a deficiency of either one has a significant effect on the metabolism of the other

- **Increased** in renal failure, dehydration, hypothyroidism, Addison's disease, adrenalectomy, severe diabetic acidosis, overuse of Mg-containing antacids.

- **Decreased** in chronic diarrhea, hemodialysis, chronic renal disease, cirrhosis, diuretic abuse, severe burns, inflammatory bowel disease, hyperaldosteronism, toxemia of pregnancy, hyperthyroidism, excessive loss of body fluids, malabsorption syndromes, chronic alcoholism, prolonged gastric drainage, long-term hyperalimentation.

- **Clinical aspects**

Problem	Subjective	Objective	Emergency Rx
Hypermagnesemia	Lethargy, flushing, nausea, vomiting, slurred speech, drowsiness, respiratory depression	Weak or absent deep tendon reflexes; prolonged PR and QT intervals, widened QRS, bradycardia; hypotension	Calcium salts; dialysis; withhold sources of Mg^{2+} excess
Hypomagnesemia	Muscle tremors, twitching, tetany, anorexia, nausea, vomiting, lethargy, insomnia	May cause unexplained hypocalcemia and hypokalemia; hyperactive deep tendon reflexes; prolonged PR and QT intervals; broad, flat T waves; PVC, VT/VF, torsade de pointes	Restriction of stimuli; administration of magnesium salts

Blood sugar (BS)

- Glucose formed from carbohydrate digestion and conversion of glycogen to glucose by the liver.

- Insulin and glucagon directly regulate the BS level. Glucagon → glycogen breakdown and causes the BS to rise; insulin increases the cell membrane permeability to glucose, transports glucose into the cells, and stimulates glycogen formation reducing BS levels.

- **Increased** in diabetes mellitus, Cushing's disease, acute emotional or physical stress, pheochromocytoma, pituitary adenoma (increased secretion of growth hormone), pancreatitis, brain trauma, chronic liver disease, chronic renal disease, pregnancy.

- **Decreased** in insulinoma, adrenal insufficiency, hypopituitarism, starvation, liver damage (especially alcoholism), premature infant, enzyme deficiency diseases, insulin overdose.

- **Glycosylated hemoglobin (HbA1C)** – indicates the average blood sugar levels for the 2 to 3 month period before the test. Helpful for evaluating treatment of diabetes. Normals vary by method test done.

Blood urea nitrogen (BUN)

- Urea (formed in the liver) and CO_2 are the final products of protein metabolism.

- The amount of urea excreted varies directly with dietary protein intake; excretion is increased in fever, diabetes, and with increased activity of the adrenal glands.

- Less sensitive than creatinine clearance for renal failure.

- **Increased (azotemia)** in impaired renal function, congestive heart failure (decreased renal perfusion), salt and water depletion, shock, GI hemorrhage (protein catabolism), acute MI, stress, excessive protein intake.

- **Decreased** in liver failure, acromegaly, malnutrition, use of anabolic steroids, over hydration, malabsorption, SIADH.

Creatinine (Cr)

▶ A byproduct of muscle creatine phosphate (used in energy metabolism); produced at a constant rate, depending on the muscle mass of the person; removed by the kidneys.

▶ **Increased** in impaired renal function, obstruction of the urinary tract, muscle disease (acromegaly, myasthenia gravis, muscular dystrophy, polio), congestive heart failure, shock, dehydration, rhabdomyolysis.

▶ **Decreased** in small stature, decreased muscle mass, severe liver disease, inadequate dietary protein intake; generally decreases in Cr are **not** clinically significant.

▶ **BUN/Cr ratio** – may be helpful in determining causes of elevations; in **prerenal azotemia** with hypoperfusion of the kidneys but <u>intact tubular function</u> (hypovolemia, congestive heart failure, ascites), the BUN is usually greater than 10X the creatinine [BUN 25 Cr 2.0) versus **renal azotemia** (true renal failure) where the ratio is usually le [BUN 25 Cr 7.0].

Uric acid

▶ Formed from the breakdown of purines in nucleic acids (adenine and guanine in RNA and DNA); 2/3 of uric acid produced daily is excreted by the kidneys; the remaining 1/3 excreted in stool.

▶ In the hospitalized patient, renal failure is the most common cause of elevations.

▶ **Increased** in gout, renal failure, alcoholism, dehydration, leukemia, lymphoma, starvation, toxemia of pregnancy, following excessive cell destruction (chemotherapy, radiation treatment, critical illness [see below]).

▶ **Decreased** in Wilson's disease, SIADH, heavy metal poisoning, Hodgkins disease, multiple myeloma, xanthinuria (deficiency of xanthine oxidase).

▶ May need to give prophylactic allopurinol prior to chemotherapy or large scale radiotherapy.

▶ **NOTE:** In the final step of purine metabolism, hypoxanthine may be converted to uric acid, free radical-containing molecules, or both. Both steps are catalyzed by the same enzyme – xanthine oxidase. Elevated levels of uric acid may indicate on-going tissue damage (e.g., critical illness). Dying cells release their DNA and RNA – the purine portions (adenine and guanine) are converted to uric acid, free radicals, or both. Much recent data suggests that elevated uric acid levels in sick patients is an independent predictor of a bad prognosis – the main reason for this is that when more uric acid is made, so are more free radicals.. Allopurinol (Zyloprim®) blocks xanthine oxidase, which is why the drug is effective in gout. It also blocks the formation of free radicals and has been shown to reduce mortality in critically-ill patients. This is illustrated in the figure below:

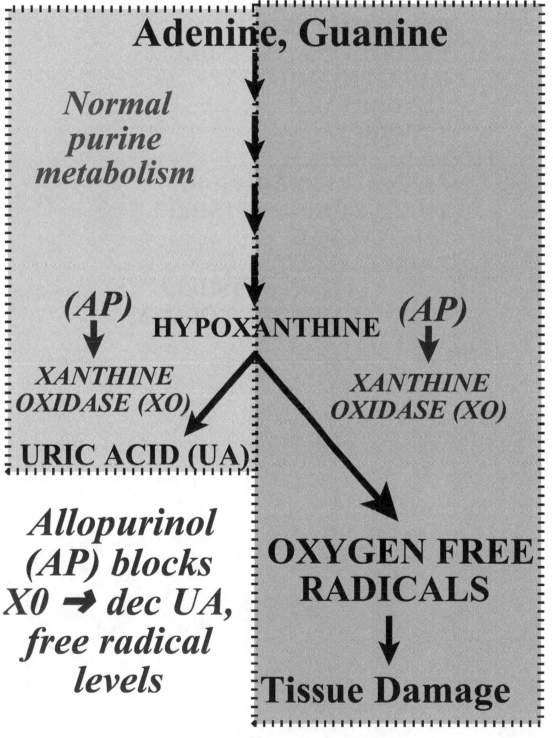

CHAPTER 5 – LIVER FUNCTION AND THYROID TESTS

LIVER FUNCTION TESTS

PARAMETERS MEASURED
THE TEST IN A "NUTSHELL"
NORMAL VALUES
PANIC VALUES
RESULTS IN A "NUTSHELL"
BASIC PHYSIOLOGY
TEST DETAILS
JAUNDICE

THYROID TESTS

PARAMETERS MEASURED
THE TEST IN A "NUTSHELL"
NORMAL VALUES
PANIC VALUES
RESULTS IN A "NUTSHELL"
SUMMARY OF PHYSIOLOGY
TEST DETAILS

CHAPTER 5 – LIVER FUNCTION AND THYROID TESTS

LIVER FUNCTION TESTS

- **Parameters measured:** Albumin, ammonia (NH_4), bilirubin (total, direct, indirect, alanine transaminase (ALT/SGPT), alkaline phosphatase (ALP), aspartate transaminase (AST, SGOT), gamma-glutamyltransferase (GGT), lactic acid dehydrogenase (LDH), total protein

- **The test in a "nutshell":** Measures various functions of the liver (e.g., storage, synthesis, bile production). Commonly ordered to evaluate jaundice, weight loss, abdominal pain, alcohol abuse.

- **Normal values:**

Parameter	Normal value (adults)
Albumin	3.8-5.0 g/dl
Ammonia (NH_4)	9-33 umol/L
Bilirubin, total	0.2-1.0 mg/dl
Bilirubin, direct (conjugated)	0.0-0.2 mg/dl
Bilirubin, indirect (unconjugated)	0.2-0.8 mg/dl
Alanine transaminase (ALT, SGPT [serum glutamic-pyruvic transaminase])	7-56 U/L
Alkaline phosphatase (ALP)	17-142 IU/L
Aspartate transaminase (AST; serum glutamic-oxaloacetic transaminase [SGOT])	5-40 U/L
Gamma-glutamyltransferase (GGT)	5-85 U/L (males); 5-55 U/L (females)
Lactic acid dehydrogenase (LDH)	313-618 U/L
Total protein	6.0-8.0 g/dl

PANIC VALUES!!

Bilirubin (in adults) > 12 mg/dl
Bilirubin (in newborns) > 15 mg/dl (kernicterus)

■ **Results in a "nutshell":**

PARAMETER	IMPLICATIONS
Albumin	Reflect state of hydration (increase with dehydration), cellular protein synthesis, kidney, and liver function.
Ammonia (NH₄)	Inc in Reye's syndrome, severe liver disease (e.g., cirrhosis, hepatic coma), GI bleeding, shock; dec in hyperornithinemia (rare metabolic disorder).
Bilirubin (total, direct [conjugated], indirect [unconjugated])	Evaluates liver function, hemolytic anemia, and newborn jaundice; inc with hepatic dysfunction, blockage of hepatobiliary tree (stone, tumor), and hemolysis.
Alanine transaminase (ALT, SGPT [serum glutamic-pyruvic transaminase])	Useful to differentiate between hemolytic jaundice and jaundice caused by liver disease; inc in parenchymal liver disease; correlates with hepatitis B virus core antigen; persons with elevations should **not** donate blood.
Alkaline phosphatase (ALP)	A tumor marker and an index of liver and bone disease; rises in proportion to new bone cell production (osteoblastic activity with deposit of calcium in the bones) or with obstruction in the biliary tract.
Aspartate transaminase (AST; serum glutamic-oxaloacetic transaminase [SGOT])	Used predominantly to indicate liver disease; was used in past (no longer in most centers) to assess acute MI.
Lactic acid dehydrogenase (LDH)	A nonspecific test sometimes helpful in confirming MI, pulmonary infarction, muscular dystrophy, and some tumors; isoenzymes may be more helpful.

Gamma-glutamyltransferase (GGT)	Very sensitive early indicator of liver disease (e.g., tumor, alcoholic hepatitis, obstructive jaundice).
Total protein	Reflects state of hydration as well as synthetic function of liver.

■ **Basic physiology**

The hepatic-portal system

▸ **Definition** – vascular system that begins with capillary beds in the viscera and ends up in the sinusoidal capillaries in the liver with no pumping mechanism (e.g., the heart) in between.

▸ **Anatomy** – major vein is the **hepatic portal vein** formed by the union of the **superior mesenteric vein** and the **splenic vein**. Each of these receives branches from various portions of the intestines as follows:

> **Hepatic portal**
> **Superior mesenteric**
> **Splenic**
> > *Inferior mesenteric*
> > *Pancreatic*
> > *Gastroepiploic*
> **Gastric**
> **Cystic**

The hepatic portal vein progressively branches, ending with the **sinusoidal capillaries** in the liver. Blood from the sinusoids is collected into **central veins** which then empty into **hepatic veins**. These eventually join the **inferior vena cava**.

▸ **Function** – nutrients absorbed from the intestines are taken to the liver to be metabolized and/or detoxified (certain drugs, waste products).

Normal functions of the liver

If we consider the normal functions of the liver, it's easy to see what happens when dysfunction is present. Most of these abnormalities translate into definable laboratory abnormalities. The main functions of the liver are listed below – laboratory implications are noted in *italics*.

61

▸ **Bile production**

- 600-1000 ml per day
- Dilutes and neutralizes stomach acid
- Emulsifies fats
- Contains bilirubin

Abnormalities result in increases of serum bilirubin levels.

▸ **Storage**

- Sugar as glycogen
- Fat
- Vitamins
- Copper
- Iron

Abnormalities result in hypoglycemia, copper storage diseases (Wilson's disease), iron storage disease (hemochromatosis)

▸ **Nutrient interconversion**

- Phospholipid production
- Hydroxylation of vitamin D (kidney also does; double process)

Abnormalities may result in malnutrition, vitamin D deficiency

▸ **Detoxification**

- Ammonia waste products
- Drugs (phenobarbital)

Abnormalities may result in elevated serum drug levels or hepatic coma (elevated ammonia levels).

▸ Phagocytosis (Kupffer cells) – *abnormalities may result in infection*

▸ Synthesis

- Albumins
- Fibrinogen
- Globulins
- Clotting proteins

Abnormalities may result in edema, immunodeficiency, or (most commonly) bleeding problems; with associated hepatocellular damage (e.g., hepatitis, cirrhosis) the SGOT, SGPT, alkaline phosphatase, and often, bilirubin levels will be abnormally high.

■ **Test details**

Albumin

▸ Regulates oncotic pressure

▸ **Increased** with IV infusions, dehydration.

▸ **Decreased** with decreased protein synthesis states (liver disease, alcoholism, malabsorption syndromes, Chrohn's disease, starvation), increased albumin loss (nephrotic syndrome, third-degree burns), poor nutrition, inadequate iron intake

Ammonia (NH$_4$)

▸ End product of protein metabolism

▸ Formed by bacteria acting on intestinal proteins + hydrolysis of glutamine in the kidneys

▸ Normally removed by liver via portal circulation and converted to urea

▸ Urea excreted by the kidneys

▸ Elevated levels affect acid-base balance and brain function significantly

▸ Does not reflect degree of hepatic coma

▸ Levels vary with protein intake

Bilirubin

▸ Byproduct of hemoglobin breakdown by RE (reticuloendothelial) system; removed from body by liver and excreted into bile.

▸ Only small amounts usually found in blood.

▸ Level rises if there is excessive destruction of RBCs or if liver unable to excrete normal amounts produced.

► Normal total level rules out any significant impairment of hepatic excretory function or excessive hemolysis; inc unconjugated more common with hemolysis; inc conjugated more likely in dysfunction or blockage of the liver/hepatobiliary tract (e.g., stone, tumor). Breakdown of total, direct, and indirect only necessary when total elevated.

► Causes of elevations with jaundice (total > 2.5 mg/dl for jaundice to appear):

Mechanism	Causes
Hepatocellular jaundice (injury or disease of the parenchymal cells of the liver	Viral hepatitis, cirrhosis, infectious mononucleosis, drugs (e.g., chlorpromazine)
Obstructive jaundice	Obstruction of common bile or hepatic ducts by stones (choledocholithiasis) or neoplasms (e.g., cancer of head of the pancreas); produces high, conjugated levels
Hemolytic (overproduction of bilirubin as a result of hemolysis; leads to high unconjugated levels)	Hemolytic disease of the newborn, any hemolytic anemia, pernicious anemia, sickle cell anemia, transfusion reactions, Crigler-Najjar syndrome (congenital lack of enzyme needed for conjugation), trauma with a large hematoma, hemorrhagic pulmonary infarction

Alanine transaminase (ALT, SGPT [serum glutamic-pyruvic transaminase])

► Occurs in high concentrations in the liver; low concentrations in heart, muscle, and kidney

► ALT doesn't always increase in acute MI (versus AST [SGOT] which often does); usually increased more than AST in acute extrahepatic biliary obstruction; less sensitive than AST to alcoholic liver disease

► **Increased in**: hepatocellular disease, active cirrhosis, metastatic liver tumor, obstructive jaundice, hepatitis, infectious mononucleosis, pancreatitis, MI, polymyositis, severe burns, trauma to skeletal muscle, severe shock.

Alkaline phosphatase (ALP)

► Originates in bone, liver, and placenta

► Functions best at a pH of 9

- Age and sex dependent; greatly increased in persons < 20 years old; males >> females until adulthood (age 21)

- **Increased** in liver disease (e.g., obstructive jaundice, liver tumors, cirrhosis, hepatitis), bone disease (Paget's disease, metastatic bone tumor. osteogenic sarcoma, osteomalacia [**not** increased in osteoporosis], celiac sprue, renal disorders), various other conditions (hyperparathyroidism, pulmonary and myocardial infarctions, cancer of lung or pancreas, ulcerative colitis, sarcoidosis, perforation of bowel, chronic renal failure, sepsis).

- **Decreased** in malnutrition, hypothyroidism, pernicious anemia, scurvy.

- An accompanying test, **5'-nucleotidase**, is elevated in the face of liver disease; elevations of ALP with a normal 5'-nucleotidase suggests bone disease.

Aspartate transaminase (AST; serum glutamic-oxaloacetic transaminase [SGOT])

- Present in tissues of high metabolic activity (liver, heart, skeletal muscle, kidney, brain, pancreas, spleen, lungs).

- Released into the circulation from the death or damage of any cells in highly metabolic tissues, regardless of the underlying disease.

- Amount of AST in the blood is directly related to # of damaged cells and the time passed between injury and obtaining the test.

- Following cell damage, AST level rises in 12 hours and stays elevated for about 5 days.

- Causes of **increased** AST levels:

Type of disease	Examples
Liver disease	Acute hepatitis, chronic hepatitis, active cirrhosis, primary or metastatic carcinoma, alcoholic hepatitis, Reye's syndrome
Myocardial infarction	Nonspecific and **should not** be relied upon for diagnosis; reaches a peak in 24 hours and returns to normal by the 3rd or 4th day.
Other	Acute pancreatitis, trauma of skeletal muscle, heat stroke, trichinosis, brain trauma, muscular dystrophy, pulmonary emboli, gangrene, malignant hyperthermia, mushroom poisoning

▸ **Decreased** AST levels occur in renal failure (azotemia) and in patients on chronic renal dialysis.

Lactic acid dehydrogenase (LDH)

▸ Widely distributed intracellular enzyme (kidney, heart, skeletal muscle, brain, liver, lungs).

▸ Increases indicate cellular death and leakage of the enzyme from cells.

▸ **Increased** in MI, pulmonary infarction, congestive heart failure, liver disease (cirrhosis, hepatitis), cancer, hypothyroidism, muscular dystrophy. Also increased in megaloblastic and pernicious anemia.

▸ **Decreased** with good response to cancer chemotherapy.

▸ **Isoenzymes** usually more helpful than LDH, by itself, since it is so ubiquitous. Normal values are (expressed as a percentage of total):

LDH1 17-27% – found in heart and red blood cells
LDH2 29-39% – found in heart and red blood cells
LDH3 19-27% – found in a variety of organs
LDH4 8-16% – found in a variety of organs
LDH5 6-16% – found in liver and skeletal muscle

An LDH "flip" (when LDH1 > LDH2) is strongly suggestive of acute MI; increases in LDH5 are common in liver disease and CHF. [**NOTE**: hemolytic anemia can also raise the percentage of LDH1, leading to an LDH "flip" identical to that seen in MI]

Gamma-glutamyltransferase (GGT)

▸ Liver is source of normal serum activity despite GGT's presence in kidney, prostate, and spleen; men have higher levels due to prostate.

▸ Very sensitive to the amount of alcohol consumed by chronic drinkers; used to monitor cessation or reduction of ETOH consumption.

▸ Elevated in all forms of liver disease and much more sensitive than either AST or ALT.

▸ **Increased** in liver disease (e.g., hepatitis, cirrhosis, carcinoma, cholestasis, mononucleosis), pancreatic disease (pancreatitis, cancer), hyperthyroidism.
▸ **Decreased** in hypothyroidism.

- **Normal** in bone disorders, pregnancy, skeletal muscle disease, strenuous exercise, and renal failure.

Total protein

- Serum proteins are a source of nutrition, a buffer system, immunoglobulins, carrier proteins, regulatory proteins, and hormones.

- Helpful to evaluate nephrotic syndromes, liver disease, and immune dysfunction; also for nutritional status in edematous and malnourished patients.

- **Increased** in dehydration and hemoconcentration stated secondary to fluid loss (e.g., vomiting, diarrhea, poor kidney function); other diseases (liver disease, multiple myeloma, sarcoidosis, collagen vascular disease, chronic inflammation, chronic infections.

- **Decreased** in starvation or malabsorption, severe liver disease and alcoholism, kidney disease (nephrotic syndrome), diarrhea, severe skin diseases and burns, severe hemorrhage, heart failure, hypothyroidism, prolonged immobilization (e.g., trauma, orthopedic surgery).

Jaundice *(enrichment)*[1]

The biochemistry of bilirubin, urobilinogen, and their interrelationship with liver function tests (LFTs) is confusing, if not downright threatening, to many of us. When I originally prepared my Lab Tests course, I asked myself a simple question: "What are the kinetics of bilirubin and where does urobilinogen come from?" Of the nearly 600,000 students I've asked, few would feel comfortable trying to answer the question, including "yours truly!" I figured that the solution must lie in my friendly collection of medical, nursing, lab, and allied health professions books. Was I ever wrong. I couldn't find the whole picture nicely summarized in any single volume I searched. After about a week, I finally put this material together — I'm very proud of it, though also quite frustrated that my thousands of dollars worth of reference books were basically worthless in this endeavor. Hopefully, you'll have the opportunity to "get it right" the first time, and understand this elegant system so you'll remember it forever.

What are the normal metabolic functions of the liver? The liver plays a major role in the metabolism of carbohydrates, fat, and proteins. In carbohydrate metabolism it:

1. Stores large quantities of glycogen.
2. Converts galactose and fructose to glucose.
3. Acts as the primary site for gluconeogenesis.

Most cells of the body play a role in fat metabolism, though the liver has a primary role in:

1. Oxidation of fats to acetyl-coenzyme A (acetyl-CoA).
2. Synthesis of cholesterol, phospholipids, and lipoproteins.
3. Fat synthesis from carbohydrates and proteins.

The liver is vital in numerous steps of protein metabolism. These include:

- Deamination of amino acids — amino acids cannot be used for energy or converted into carbohydrates or fats until they have been deaminated (ammonia removed).

- Formation of urea — large amounts of ammonia are formed during the deamination process, as well as produced by the metabolism of protein by colonic bacteria. The liver converts ammonia to urea, which is then excreted in the urine.

- Formation of plasma proteins — all plasma proteins, except for gamma globulins, are made in the liver. Gamma globulins are made in the lymphoid tissues.

- Metabolism of amino acids and synthesis of compounds from amino acids — the liver synthesizes nonessential amino acids and converts all the amino acids into other metabolically significant compounds.

Other functions of the liver include:

- Storage of vitamins and iron.
- Production of clotting factors II, VII, IX, and X.
- Detoxification and excretion of drugs and hormones.
- Conjugation and secretion of bilirubin into the bile.

My jaundiced opinion. Jaundice is common in a wide variety of disease states. For now, we'll limit ourselves to adults with all of their "innards" intact. Neonatal jaundice, hereditary conjugation defects, asplenia, and persons without a gallbladder make the picture more confusing than it needs to be.

Basic facts ("simple yet true!"). In this section, I want to outline a simple but elegant pathophysiologically-based approach to the "yellow fellow" — a patient with clinical jaundice. The bottom line is simple, but to understand, rather than memorize, I respectfully *beg* you to follow the steps, and not jump ahead. Just so you don't lose any precious sleep, I'll mention that the "bottom line" is "Give 'em a cup. . . " When we're done with the details, the beauty of this will *prove* to you that the dip UA is the single *best* liver function test in a jaundiced patient!

This approach is based on certain facts:

1. Red blood cells (RBCs) live 120 days; at that time they undergo a normal apoptotic (genetically-programmed) death. Dead RBCs are then "recycled" by the reticuloendothelial system (RES), primarily the tissue macrophages and spleen.

> **REMEMBER**: The bilirubin system is a *normal* excretory mechanism for hemoglobin breakdown products. Jaundice is seen during a *normal response* to an *abnormal situation*.

2. When RBCs are recycled by the RES, hemoglobin is broken down into its constituents, heme and globin.

3. Globin is a vital plasma protein and is recycled to the protein pool of the body.

4. Heme is broken down and prepared for excretion. First, iron is removed and "recycled" by binding to transferrin (iron transport protein). This replenishes the body's iron stores and provides iron for new hemoglobin synthesis. Interestingly, carbon monoxide (CO) is made in the process and acts as a chemical messenger, causing the conversion of GTP to cyclic GMP (cGMP). CO is then excreted in the lungs. The remnants of heme are then eliminated from the body (described in detail immediately below).

5. The entire purpose of the bilirubin system is to *eliminate* heme from the body via a series of metabolic steps.

The main reason people get confused is because they lose track of the reason for the entire system — to *metabolize* heme and *eliminate* it in either the stool (first choice) or the urine (second choice).

The "bilirubin factory tour." It's easiest to separate out the steps in space and time, though we all know that *in vivo*, there is some overlap. The areas of our "factory" are: **[Figure]**

> ***REMEMBER***: The main purpose of the bilirubin system is to *metabolize* heme and *eliminate* it in either the stool (first choice) or in the urine (second choice).

1. The "mortuary" — the reticuloendothelial system, primarily tissue macrophages and the spleen is essentially a mortician, preparing the dead RBC for recycling and excretion of non-recyclabl components (e.g., heme).

2. The "conjugator" — the liver; converts heme into an excretable form.

3. The "excretor" — the GI tract and kidneys.

HEMOGLOBIN BREAKDOWN

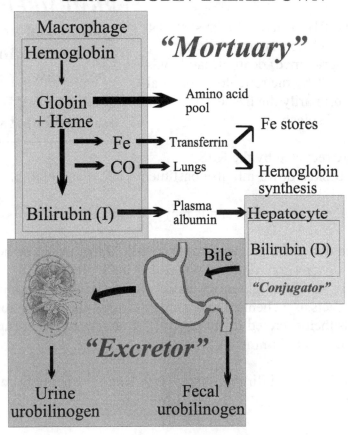

Figure — The "Bilirubin Factory Tour"

Of course, all three sections of the bilirubin "factory" are interconnected by blood vessels. In a nutshell, the process goes something like this:

1.   The RES recycles iron and globin, and converts heme to a nonwater-soluble form of bilirubin.

2.   The liver conjugates nonwater-soluble bilirubin to a water-soluble form so it can be secreted into the bile.

3.   Bile drains into the duodenum via the common bile duct; bilirubin "hitchhikes" along.

4.   Bilirubin is converted to "urobilinogens" in the colon, and either excreted in the stool or filtered by the kidneys and excreted in the urine.

5.   Either way, the end product of heme breakdown, urobilinogens, are excreted from the body.

Now, let's observe the process in more detail and add in the many names for the two forms of bilirubin. Like it or not, this is potentially confusing, so watch out — you and I didn't create this mess, we just have to deal with it!

PART I: In the "mortuary" (RES). The RES sequesters the dead RBCs, and enzymes break down their cell walls. Hemoglobin is separated into globin, which is recycled into the plasma protein pool, and heme (an iron-containing protoporphyrin, for those of you *really interested* in biochemistry), which must be prepared for excretion. Iron from heme is recycled by binding to transferrin in an energy-requiring reaction that also produces carbon monoxide (CO). CO is excreted via the lungs.

The RES converts heme to **biliverdin**, then to **unconjugated bilirubin**. The latter, an early form of bilirubin, is not water-soluble. (Though I strongly believe that the only two terms for bilirubin should be "water-soluble" and "nonwater-soluble," it's a battle I won't win.)
Early, nonwater-soluble bilirubin goes by one of two names, depling on the laboratory — **unconjugated** or **indirect**. Remember, the whole purpose of our tour is to see how *early, nonwater-soluble (i.e., unconjugated, indirect) bilirubin is made water-soluble so it will dissolve in bile to be excreted into the GI tract and eliminated from the body*! Pretty straightforward, eh?

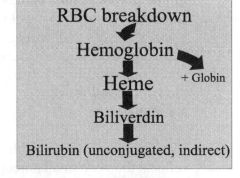

The "yellow taxi" ride to the liver. Bilirubin is converted to a water-soluble form in the liver, but first it needs to get there. Remember that this early form isn't going to dissolve by itself in the blood (nonwater-soluble). To get to the liver, via the blood, unconjugated bilirubin (which we'll abbreviate as BU) binds to albumin (BU-A). This is a common way that nonwater-soluble molecules become temporarily soluble in liquid. Albumin acts as the "yellow taxi" and carries BU to the liver. Like any good cab driver, the albumin taxi drops BU off and returns to the cab stand (plasma) to await further passengers. Don't forget — we *still* want to get rid of BU, regardless of what name we call it.

When we measure unconjugated (indirect) bilirubin levels in the lab, we're essentially determining how many "passengers" (BU) are in "yellow taxis" on their way to the liver to be conjugated. In more formal terms, the unconjugated bilirubin test measured albumin-bound unconjugated bilirubin levels. Keep this in mind, and consider which non-hepatic problem would lead to jaundice and an elevation of indirect (early, nonwater-soluble, etc.) bilirubin. The answer in a bit. . .

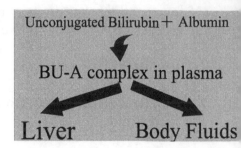

PART II: In the "converter" (liver). The hepatocyte performs two separate, though related, actions of early, nonwater-soluble bilirubin (BU). The first is **conjugation**, the process of chemically adding two glucuronide molecules, resulting in the formation of **bilirubin diglucuronide** (BRG). BRG is a long word, so I find it easier to call it "late," or water-soluble, bilirubin. The lab people use somewhat different terms — **conjugated** or **direct**. So, the liver conjugates BU to a water-soluble form. Second, the hepatocyte then *secretes* the conjugated (direct, late, water-soluble) bilirubin, via the bile canaliculi, into the biliary drainage system (i.e., bile ducts, hepatic ducts, gallbladder).

> **REMEMBER**: Once early bilirubin (nonwater-soluble, indirect, unconjugated) reaches the liver, it *will* be converted to late bilirubin (water-soluble, direct, conjugated).

It's important to understand that conjugation and secretion, though both carried out by the hepatocyte, are *separate* processes. As such, various diseases may damage one function (e.g., secretion) but leave the other (e.g., conjugation) intact. In fact, this is usually the case. Conjugation isn't completely impaired until late hepatic failure — by then, the patient has "flapping" (sign language for "I need a transplant") and numerous other stigmata of severe liver failure. Secretion, on the other hand, is impaired (but seldom completely blocked) at a much earlier stage. Diseases causing hepatocellular damage, such as hepatitis, will affect *secretion* and rarely alter *conjugation* unless they progress to end-stage liver failure. In most cases, it's safe to assume that once unconjugated bilirubin (early, nonwater-soluble, indirect) reaches the liver, it *will* be converted to conjugated bilirubin (late, water-soluble, direct).

The *conjugated* (*direct*) bilirubin level that we measure in the lab reflects the very small amount of conjugated bilirubin that "backs up" normally in the serum. The *total bilirubin* level is the mathematical sum of unconjugated plus conjugated (indirect + direct) bilirubin levels. Most experts recommend that you measure only two of the three, and calculate the remaining value. If you rely on separate lab tests to measure each, the math never works out, and outside reviewers have a picnic!

72

PART III: The "hitchhiker." Once in the bile, conjugated bilirubin flows through the sphincter of Odi into the duodenum. Bilirubin has *no* digestive functions; it's merely a passive follower, or "hitchhiker," taking the shortest direct and "physiologically-legal" route to the intestine. Remember — our body's "mission" is to excrete heme!

In the intestines. Water-soluble bilirubin passes through the duodenum and small intestine unchanged. In the colon, normal enteric bacteria convert it to **urobilinogens (UBs)**, the final breakdown product of heme and the form in which "heme" is finally excreted normally (at last!). Most of the urobilinogen mixes with fecal material, imparting the normal brownish color of stool to it. Some physiologists refer to this portion of urobilinogen as stercobilin. Thus (and this is gross, but memorable!), urobilinogen (stercobilin) is essentially "brown dye #2." It passes in the stool and is eliminated from the body, which is what we wanted to do in the first place — right?

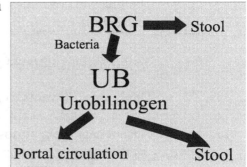

NOTE: Some experts use the term "urobilinogens" as a generic term for conjugated bilirubin broken down by the colonic bacteria. Others use stercobilin *to refer to the portion that "colors" the stool, and* urobilinogen *as the remnant that is excreted in the urine and lends a golden hue to the urine color. The concept of elimination of bilirubin breakdown products, first in the stool, then in the urine (if any is left over) is more important than specific names. The term "urobilinogens" will work for both — and the "bottom line" is unchanged, since the dip UA indeed measures "urobilinogen" in the urine, as well as bilirubin. For simplicity's sake, I use the term "urobilinogens" to refer to both compounds, regardless of their location in the stool or urine.*

In the "beans" (kidneys). The quanity of urobilinogens that leave the body in the stool is dependent on the bilirubin load thrust upon the liver. If there is more unconjugated bilirubin than usual to conjugate, more conjugated bilirubin is made. More enters the intestine and more urobilinogens are made by the colonic flora. Remember, regardless of the amount, we *still* want to excrete urobilinogens from the body.

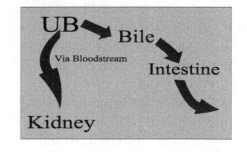

The urobilinogen that doesn't pass in the stool is reabsorbed into the blood (portal circulation) and transported to the kidneys. Being water-soluble, it freely crosses the glomerular filtration membrane and is excreted in the urine. Normally, the dip urinalysis (UA) contains "zero to trace" urobilinogen, because most is excreted in the stool. Whatever appears in the urine represents the "colonic overload" that wasn't excreted via the stool. So, the "beans" are the "back door" or secondary route for final heme breakdown product excretion.

Make certain you're comfortable at this stage that:

1.   Colonic bacteria manufacture urobilinogens from conjugated bilirubin.

2.   Urobilinogens "color" the stools brown, and to some extent, the urine yellow.

3.   If there is complete hepatobiliary obstruction (e.g., common duct stone, pancreatic cancer, choledochal cyst), *no bilirubin* enters the GI tract.

4.   If there is *no bilirubin* in the gut, there can be *no urobilinogen* made by the colonic bacteria.

5.   The presence of *any* urobilinogen in the urine virtually excludes *complete* hepatobiliary obstruction.

6.   Stool without "brown dye #2" can't be normal color.

7.   The body *still* wants to get rid of the bilirubin!

I know these tenets seem almost insultingly simple — trust me, and NOT because I'm a doctor. As obvious as they may seem during a casual reading, most students lose sight of this simple elegance at some point.

The meaning of jaundice. The presence of clinical jaundice means that a patient's serum *total* bilirubin level is elevated (usually 2.5 - 3.0 mg/dL). This is true regardless of whether the elevation consists primarily of conjugated, unconjugated, or (rarely) both types of bilirubin. In fact, we could argue that measuring the actual total bilirubin level in adults, other than to follow a patient's progress, is academic.

In adults, the absolute "peak" of the bilirubin level isn't as much of a concern as it is in newborns. Bilirubin doesn't cross the blood-brain barrier, which is fully developed in adults. So, the risk of kernicterus and brain damage is absent. We could argue that once we visually observe jaundice, we *already know* that the total bilirubin level is up. Remember — once you see yellow, you already *know* the bilirubin level is "too high." In fact, we can often predict from the dip UA which fraction (direct or indirect) predominates.

Generically speaking, there are only two causes of jaundice (if we exclude congenital conjugation defects) — hemolysis or "liverolysis." Intravascular hemolysis is *not* a liver problem and requires a totally different lab and clinical approach than does "liverolysis." Of course, I invented the term "liverolysis," yet the concept is very helpful. Once we've determined that the patient has "liver jaundice," we can use our understanding of bilirubin kinetics to differentiate between the two types of liver problems — **obstructive jaundice** (e.g., common duct stone, pancreatic tumor) and **hepatocellular jaundice** (e.g., hepatitis, toxins such as carbon tetrachloride, acetaminophen, or alcohol).

Liver problems, regardless of whether primarily obstructive or destructive (hepatocellular injury), result in a backup of conjugated bilirubin in the blood. Though the causes are different for each type of jaundice, the bottom line effect is the same. The backup causes jaundice and an elevation of the serum total and direct bilirubin levels. Remember that the body *still* wants to get rid of bilirubin (heme) — what doesn't get to the bowel (due to failure of hepatic secretion or due to hepatobiliary obstruction) is excreted in the urine. Thus, the appearance of bilirubin in the urine *always* means a liver problem — either obstruction or "destruction."

What are the common causes of* unconjugated *hyperbilirubinemia? There are three generic causes of unconjugated hyperbilirubinemia:

1.   Bilirubin overproduction — excessive hemolysis of red blood cells or resorption of major hemorrhages are the most common.

2.   Reduced hepatic uptake of bilirubin formed peripherally — Gilbert syndrome (see number 3); drugs (rifampin).

3.   Impaired hepatic conjugation of bilirubin — neonatal jaundice; Crigler-Najjar syndrome (congenital decrease or absence of bilirubin uridine duiphosphate-glucuronosyltransferase (UGT); Gilbert syndrome (congenital mutation in the UGT gene resulting in mild, fluctuating unconjugated hyperbilirubinemia).

What are the common causes of* conjugated *hyperbilirubinemia? Three common causes are:

1.   Dubin-Johnson syndrome — congenital defect resulting in defective secretion of bilirubin due to absence of canalicular plasma transport protein.

2.   Rotor syndrome — asymptomatic, genetic form of conjugated hyperbilirubinemia.

3.   Cholestasis — due to hepatocellular dysfunction (failure of hepatocyte secretion of bile) or biliary obstruction.

A simplified (and still correct) approach. If we exclude neonatal jaundice and congenital defects (e.g., Dubin-Johnson, Gilbert syndromes) the causes of jaundice boil down to two: increased bilirubin production or decreased bilirubin excretion. By "excretion," I mean failure of conjugated bilirubin to reach the bowel and undergo conversion to urobilinogen.

Decreased bilirubin excretion occurs due to some type of hepatobiliary dysfunction, either hepatocellular damage ("destruction," with failure of the hepatocyte to secrete bile into the ductal system) or obstruction (partial or complete). Either results in an accumulation of *conjugated* bilirubin.

The only cause of increased bilirubin production is intravascular hemolysis. And, this results in an increased level of *unconjugated* bilirubin, which is then metabolized normally.

75

Obstructive jaundice. Let's assume that the entire system works well until we get to the common bile duct. Mentally, let's tie it off with a nice yellow ribbon and determine what would happen. Clinically, we see this as complete obstructive jaundice due to common duct stones, tumor, cysts, or (less commonly) long-standing inflammation. Since the GI tract is "closed for business" to the liver and its ducts, no bilirubin can enter the bowel. Think about what happens at this point:

1. No conjugated bilirubin enters the intestines — it *must* back up into the blood. The patient becomes jaundiced and the elevated serum bilirubin is primarily conjugated.

2. Since there is no conjugated bilirubin entering the colon, the bacteria can't make urobilinogens. Without "brown dye #2," the stool loses its normal color, leading to acholic (clay-colored) stools. Since no urobilinogens can be made, there can't be any excess in the bowel to "back up" into the urine, can there?

3. Though obstruction has caused virtually all of the conjugated bilirubin to back up into the blood, don't lose sight of the body's primary mission — it *still* wants to get rid of the stuff. Since the usual route (GI tract) isn't available, all of the conjugated bilirubin is excreted (eliminated) in the urine. Thus, we see bilirubinuria and ***LOTS*** of it. Of course, since none of this conjugated bilirubin finds its way to the colon to be made into urobilinogen, the hint is a jaundiced patient with high urine bilirubin levels (3-4+) and *no* urobilinogen in the urine.

> ***REMEMBER***: the presence of *any* urobilinogen in the dip UA excludes complete hepatobiliary obstruction.

At that point, I recommend that the next test be a CT scan or ultrasound looking for pancreatic cancer, a common duct stone, or a choledochal cyst (cyst of the biliary tree). The only other test we might need is an ALT or AST level. In pure obstruction, these enzymes aren't usually elevated more than twice normal. The only time these ALT or AST levels rise greater than twice normal during obstruction is if there is concomitant ascending cholangitis. This is unusual and these patients are incredibly ill. Most people with purely obstructive jaundice, unless they have a common duct stone, have painless jaundice. And, even those with an impacted stone may not have pain.

Hepatocellular jaundice. "Destructive" jaundice means that the hepatocytes are injured, for any of a number of reasons. This generic process is called **hepatocellular injury**. They contain enzymes, such as ALT and AST, that are normal cellular components to catalyze day to day chemical reactions. That's why there are *normal* levels of these enzymes in the serum — this reflects normal cell turnover. Only when the hepatocytes are injured significantly do their membrane walls become abnormally permeable, allowing more enzymes to leak into the serum. Thus, elevations of ALT or AST greater than twice normal imply hepatocellular damage.

Remember that secretion of bilirubin into the bile by the hepatocyte is lost relatively *early,* but that conjugation continues until end stage hepatic failure. Patients with hepatocellular jaundice, such as hepatitis, conjugate all the indirect bilirubin that reaches the liver (as long as they don't develop end-stage hepatic failure). The problem is that they don't *secrete* it into the bile as well as they normally would. It's a safe bet that some conjugated bilirubin will back up, due to loss of hepatic secretion, and need to be excreted in the urine.

As a general rule, there is less bilirubin "backed up" in hepatocellular damage than in complete obstruction. The reason: Some conjugated bilirubin enters the bowel (since a portion is secreted normally), and some urobilinogens are made. Typically, the urine bilirubin levels are not as high as in complete obstruction. If the UA shows some bilirubin (which *must be* conjugated, since it's dissolved in the urine!), as well as urobilinogen, that patient is very unlikely to have complete biliary obstruction. Why? Of course — some bilirubin *must* have entered the colon for urobilinogen to be made and, thus, to "back up" into the urine.

Hemolytic jaundice. In intravascular hemolysis, the defect lies not in the hepatobiliary system, but in the red blood cell (RBC). Essentially, the "mortuary" is overloaded with prematurely lysed RBCs. As such, there is more heme to excrete. Assuming the rest of the system is OK (which is usually a safe assumption), all the unconjugated bilirubin that gets to the liver will be conjugated. The patient is jaundiced due to the load of early, unconjugated bilirubin taking the "yellow taxi" to the liver to be excreted. Again, regardless of the cause, don't forget that the body's "mission" is to get rid of heme! And, if we measure serum bilirubin levels, the total *and* indirect (unconjugated) fractions are elevated.

Once unconjugated reaches the liver, it is conjugated as in the normal patient. The amounts of conjugated bilirubin made are just *increased.* Not a problem, as the hepatobiliary system has great functional reserve. Once conjugated, conjugated bilirubin is secreted into the bile. In hemolysis, there is *more* than usual. Thus, the colonic bacteria make *more* urobilinogens. Since the whole purpose of the system is *still* to eliminate urobilinogens, chances are excellent that more of them will back up in the blood and require excretion by the kidneys. So, we'd expect to find elevated levels of urobilinogen in the urine, but *no* bilirubin of any kind.

The clue here is a jaundiced patient (implies elevated bilirubin), no bilirubin, but *lots* of urobilinogen in the urine. The UA is telling us that "extra" urobilinogen has overloaded the GI tract and is being eliminated via the kidneys. Since there is no backup of bilirubin, the liver must be OK. So, our conclusion — hemolysis. The next series of "tests" should involve the blood cells (e.g., Coombs, Hgb, Hct), *not* the liver.

The bottom line. By now it should be clear that of the common types of jaundice, only liver problems result in bilirubinuria; hemolysis does not. So, when you see a "yellow fellow," give him a cup — meaning obtain a dip UA. Look first for one thing — bilirubin. Remember, to appear in the urine, bilirubin must be water soluble; thus, *only* conjugated bilirubin is detectable on the dip UA. Then:

- If there is any bilirubin in the urine, you are dealing with "liverolysis."

- Large urine bilirubin levels with absolutely no urobilinogen suggest complete hepatobiliary obstruction.

- A mixed picture (some bilirubin, some urobilinogen) suggests hepatocellular damage (or partial obstruction).

- Regardless of the presence, absence, or amount of urobilinogen in the dip UA, the presence of any bilirubin means a liver problem.

- Use ALT or AST (GPT/GOT) to confirm hepatocellular damage (elevated greater than twice normal). Then you can judiciously consider the next step (e.g., hepatitis antigen testing).

- If there is no bilirubin on the dip UA, the problem is most likely hemolysis; elevated urobilinogen levels in the *absence* of bilirubin strongly support this conclusion. Congenital abnormalities of bilirubin metabolism will *not* increase the amount of urobilinogen made. Only hemolysis actually increases the "workload" on the RE system ("mortuary").

> *REMEMBER*: the main purpose of the bilirubin system is to *metabolize* heme and *eliminate* it in either the stool (first choice) or in the urine (second choice).

THYROID TESTS

- **Parameters measured:** Total T4 (T4), Free T4 (FT4), Total T3 (T3), TSH, thyroid antibodies (thyroglobulin antibodies), thyroid microsomal antibodies

- **The test in a "nutshell":** Measures the activity of the thyroid gland and its hormones, which affect virtually all metabolic processes in the body. Also helpful in detecting thyroid diseases and cancer.

- **Normal values:**

Parameter	Normal value (adults)
Total T4 (T4)	**4.6-12 ug/dl**
Free T4 (FT4)	**0.7-1.9 ng/dl**
Total T3 (T3)	**80-180 ng/dl**

TSH	0.3-5.0 mU/ml
Thyroid antibodies (thyroglobulin antibodies)	nondetectable
Thyroid microsomal antibodies (antithyroid peroxidase antibodies)	nondetectable

PANIC VALUES!!

T4 (in adults) >18.0 μg/dL
T4 (in newborns) <3.5 or >18.0 μg/dL

- **Results in a "nutshell":**

PARAMETER	IMPLICATIONS
Total T4 (T4)	Measures the concentration of thyroxine (T4) in the serum. This includes both bound and free hormone. Only the free hormone, about 0.05% of the total, is biologically active.
Free T4 (FT4)	Measures the concentration of free thyroxine, the only biologically active fraction, in the serum. Very useful in the diagnosis of hypo- or hyperthyroidism.
Total T3 (T3)	Measures the concentration of triiodothyronine (T3) in the serum. Helpful in the diagnosis of hyperthyroidism. Rarely helpful in hypothyroidism (the last test to become abnormal).
TSH	Measures the concentration of thyroid stimulating hormone in the serum. Helpful in diagnosis of both hypo- and hyperthyroidism.
Thyroid antibodies (thyroglobulin antibodies)	Inc in Hashimoto's thyroiditis (> 90% of cases), thyroid carcinoma (45% of cases), some cases of thyrotoxicosis, pernicious anemia (> 50% of cases in low titres). Up to 10% of a normal population may have low titres with no symptoms of disease.
Thyroid microsomal antibodies	Positive in Hashimoto's thyroiditis; < 10% of patients with thyroid carcinoma have positive result; positive in 99% of patients with early hypothyroidism.

- **Summary of Physiology**

  ▸ Thyroxine (T4), produced by the thyroid gland, is the major hormone controlling metabolic rate. The thyroid also produces a small amount of triiodothyroxine (T3).

  ▸ Most thyroxine is carried in the blood, bound to proteins such as thyroid binding globulin(TBG), produced by the liver. A small amount (0.05% or less) is free, biologically active and unaffected by TBG levels.

  ▸ T4 is converted into triiodothyroxine (T3) in cells where it is used in making proteins.

  ▸ Available thyroxine may be affected by thyroid disease or by other disease affecting TBG levels, such as liver or kidney disease and drugs such as the oral contraceptive pill

  ▸ The hypothalamus secretes thyrotrophin releasing hormone (TRH) which stiumulates th pituitary to release thyroid stimulating hormone (TSH). This then tells the thyroid to produce T3 and T4, which in turn feedback to suppress the release of TRH.

- **Test Details**

Total T4

  ▸ Anything that affects levels of thyroid binding globulin (TBG), albumin, or thyroid binding prealbumin (transthyretin) will affect the total thyroxine but not the free hormone.

  ▸ Estrogens and acute liver disease will increase thyroid binding, while androgens, steroids, chronic liver disease and severe illness can decrease it.

Free T4 (FT4)

  ▸ The free thyroxine is not affected by changes in concentrations of binding proteins such as TBG and thyroid binding prealbumin. Thus such conditions as pregnancy, or estroge and androgen therapy do not affect the FT4.

  ▸ Diagnosis of thyroid disease

    • The finding of an elevated TSH and low FT4 indicates primary hypothyroidism due to disease in the thyroid gland.

    • A low TSH and low FT4 indicates hypothyroidism due to a problem involving the pituitary gland.

- A low TSH with an elevated FT4 is found in individuals who have hyperthyroidism.

  ▸ **Increased levels** – acute thyroiditis, birth control pills, clofibrate, contrast x-rays using iodine, estrogen therapy, heparin, heroin, hyperthyroidism, pregnancy, thyrotoxicosis, toxic thyroid adenoma, cirrhosis, severe non-thyroid disease

  ▸ **Decreased levels** – anabolic steroids, androgens, antithyroid drugs, cretinism, hypothyroidism, kidney failure, lithium, myxedema, phenytoin, propranolol

Total T3

  ▸ This test measures both bound and free hormone. Only the free hormone is biologically active, but it is only 0.5% of the total. Anything that effects thyroid binding globulin (TBG), or albumin will effect the total triiodothyronine but not the free.

  ▸ T3 is increased in almost all cases of hyperthyroidism and usually goes up before the T4 does. Thus, the T3 is a more sensitive indicator of hyperthyroidism than the total T4.

  ▸ In hypothyroidism the T3 is often normal even when the T4 is low. Patients can be severely hypothyroid with a high TSH and low FT4 but have a normal T3.

  ▸ The T3 is decreased during acute illness and starvation, and is affected by several medications including propranolol, steroids, and amiodarone.

  ▸ **Increased levels** – T3 levels normally rise when a woman is pregnant or using birth-control pills. Elevated T3 levels can also occur in patients who use estrogen or methadone or who have hyperthyroidism, thyroiditis, T3 thyrotoxicosis, toxic adenoma.

  ▸ **Decreased levels** – acute or chronic illness, hypothyroidism, kidney or liver disease, starvation, anabolic steroids, androgens, phenytoin, propranolol, reserpine, salicylates (high doses)

TSH

  ▸ TSH is under negative feedback control by the amount of free thyroid hormone (T4 and T3) in the circulation and positive control by the hypothalamic thyroid releasing hormone (TRH).

- Hypothyroidism – in the case of primary thyroid hormone deficiency the TSH level should be elevated. The TSH alone cannot be used to screen for secondary hypothyroidism and usually requires a measurement of thyroid hormone levels to be adequately interpreted.

  - A value greater than 20 mU/ml is a good indicator of primary failure of the thyroid gland.

  - A value of between 5 and 15 is a borderline value which may require more careful evaluation.

  - If the hypothyroid state is due to failure of the pituitary gland (TSH) or the hypothalamus (TRH), the values for TSH may be low, normal or occasionally in the borderline range. The presence of low free T4 with a TSH of less than 10 strongly suggests a pituitary or hypothalamic etiology for the hypothyroidism (secondary hypothyroidism).

- Hyperthyroidism

  - Because high levels of free thyroid hormone will suppress TSH levels, in almost all case of hyperthyroidism the TSH values will be less than 0.3 and usually less the 0.1 mU/L.

  - The degree of suppression of TSH does not always reflect the severity of the hyperthyroidism; therefore a measurement of free thyroid hormone levels is usually required in patients with a suppressed TSH level.

  - If the free T4 is normal, the T3 should be checked as it is the first hormone to increase in early hyperthyroidism.

- TSH levels to monitor thyroid hormone dosing

  - High TSH levels usually indicates under-treatment, while low values usually indicate over-treatment.

  - Abnormal TSH values should be interpreted with the measurement of free thyroid hormone before modifying therapy because serum thyroid hormone levels change more quickly than TSH levels.

  - Patients who have recently been started on thyroid hormone, or who have been noncompliant until shortly before an office visit may have normal T4 and T3 levels, though their TSH levels are still elevated.

CHAPTER 6 – HEPATITIS AND AIDS TESTS
HEPATITIS TESTS
HEPATITIS A
HEPATITIS B
HEPATITIS C
HEPATITIS D
HEPATITIS E
HEPATITIS F
HEPATITIS G
AIDS TESTS
PARAMETERS MEASURED
THE TEST IN A "NUTSHELL"
NORMAL VALUES
PANIC VALUES
RESULTS IN A "NUTSHELL"
TEST DETAILS

CHAPTER 6 – HEPATITIS AND AIDS TESTS

Hepatitis tests – used to detect the presence of current or old hepatitis. The various tests that may be used currently are discussed below, and summarized in the attached tables.

- ▸ **Hepatitis A** – acquired via enteric transmission, infects the GI tract, and is eliminated through the feces; the presence of **IgM antibody to hepatitis A virus (IgM anti-HAV)** and the **total antibody to hepatitis A virus (anti-HAV)** identifies the disease.

  - **Anti-HAV IgM** – IgM antibody to hepatitis A virus; indicative of <u>recent, active infection</u> with hepatitis A virus; appears after 4-6 weeks of infection.

  - **Anti-HAV** – total antibody to hepatitis A virus; confirms <u>previous exposure and immunity</u> to hepatitis A virus; appears 8-12 weeks after infection.

Antibody	Clinical Utility
IgM anti-HAV	• Peak titres occur during the first week of clinical disease and disappear within 3-6 months • Detection of this antibody is an excellent way of diagnosing HAV
IgG anti-HAV	• Peak after one month of the disease and may persist for years • Indicates previous exposure to HAV, noninfectivity, and immunity

- ▸ **Hepatitis B** – transmitted via blood exposure (e.g., needlestick), may be sexually transmitted; central virus core contains **core antigen** and the surrounding viral envelope contains the **surface antigen**. Assessment consists of measurement of **core antigen (HbcAg)**, **envelope antigen (HbeAg)**, and **surface antigen (HbsAg)** or their corresponding antibodies.

  - **HbsAg** – hepatitis B surface antigen; appears at 4-12 weeks; indicates <u>active disease, chronic disease, or carrier state</u>; does NOT indicate past infection that has cleared.

  - **Anti-HBs** – antibody to hepatitis B surface antigen; appears at 4-10 months; when present, typically indicates <u>permanent immunity</u> (successful hepatitis B vaccination, clinical recovery from illness).

  - **IgM anti-HBc** – isolated IgM antibody against core antigen; appears at 6-14 weeks; indicates <u>acute infection</u>.

- **IgG anti-HBc** --antibody to hepatitis B core antigen; appears 6-14 weeks after infection; together with HbsAB, indicates <u>past infection and immunity</u>.
- **HBeAg** – hepatitis virus envelope antigen; appears at 4-12 weeks of infection; when present, indicates a <u>high degree of infectivity</u>.
- **Anti-HBe** – antibody to hepatitis Be antigen; appears at 8-16 weeks after infection starts; associated with <u>recovery</u>. Not helpful to indicate chronic or carrier state.

Antibody/Antigen	Clinical Utility
HBsAg	• Increased levels = first evidence of infection • Establishes infection with HBV and implies infectivity • Persistence associated with chronic hepatitis
Anti-HBs	• Specific antibody to HBsAg • Appears after disappearance of HBsAg and after successful vaccination • Signals recovery, noninfectivity, and immunity
IgM Anti-HBc	• Appears shortly after HBsAg detected • Indicates acute HBV infection • Takes 3-6 months to clear • May reappear during flares of chronic hepatitis
IgG Anti-HBc	• Appears during acute infection • Persists indefinitely
HBeAg	• Found only in HBsAg-positive serum • Indicates viral replication and infectivity • Persistence indicates increased likelihood of chronic hepatitis B • Disappearance, followed by anti-HBe signifies decreased viral replication, decreased infectivity
HBV DNA	• Parallels presence of HBeAg • A more sensitive and precise marker of viral replication and infectivity

▸ **Hepatitis C (nonA-nonB)** – transmitted parenterally; confirmed by **antibodies to hepatitis C (anti-HCV)**. These indicate <u>active disease, chronic disease, and infectivity</u>. To date, there are no known serological markers for a carrier state.

Diagnosis of acute disease can be problematic because anti-HCV is not always present when the patient develops symptoms and seeks medical care. In 30 to 40 percent of patients, anti-HCV is not detected until 2 to 8 weeks after onset of symptoms. In this situation, testing for HCV RNA is helpful, as this marker is present even before the onset of symptoms and lasts through the acute illness. Another approach to diagnosis of acute hepatitis C is to repeat the anti-HCV testing a month after onset of illness.

Test	Clinical Utility
Anti-HCV antibody	• Presence signifies infection (acute or chronic)
HCV RNA	• Presence confirms infection • Absence if anti-HCV is present suggests past infection with recovery

DETAILS ON TESTING FOR HEPATITIS C *(enrichment)*

Serologic Tests – Some patients with chronic hepatitis C have normal serum alanine aminotransferase (ALT, SGPT) levels, even when tested on multiple occasions. In this and other situations in which the diagnosis of chronic hepatitis C may be questioned, the diagnosis should be confirmed by testing for HCV RNA. The presence of HCV RNA indicates that the patient has ongoing viral infection despite normal ALT levels.

Enzyme Immunoassay – Anti-HCV is detected by enzyme immunoassay (EIA). The third-generation test (EIA-3) used today is more sensitive and specific than previous ones. However, as with all enzyme immunoassays, false-positive results are occasionally a problem with the EIA-3. Additional or confirmatory testing is often helpful.

The best approach to confirm the diagnosis of hepatitis C is to test for HCV RNA using a sensitive assay such as polymerase chain reaction (PCR) or transcription mediated amplification (TMA). The presence of HCV RNA in serum indicates an active infection.

Testing for HCV RNA is also helpful in patients in whom EIA tests for anti-HCV are unreliable. For instance, immunocompromised patients may test negative for anti-HCV despite having HCV infection because they may not produce enough antibodies for detection with EIA. Likewise, patients with acute hepatitis may test negative for anti-HCV when first tested. Antibody is present in almost all patients by 1 month after onset of acute illness; thus, patients with acute hepatitis who initially test negative may need followup testing. In these situations, HCV RNA is usually present and confirms the diagnosis.

Recombinant Immunoblot Assay – Immunoblot assays can be used to confirm anti-HCV reactivity as well. These tests are also called "Western blots"; serum is incubated on nitrocellulose strips on which four recombinant viral proteins are blotted. Color changes indicate that antibodies are adhering to the proteins. An immunoblot is considered positive if two or more proteins react and is considered indeterminate if only one positive band is detected. In some clinical situations, confirmatory testing by immunoblotting is helpful, such as for the person with anti-HCV detected by EIA who tests negative for HCV RNA. The EIA anti-HCV reactivity could represent a false-positive reaction, recovery from hepatitis C, or continued virus infection with levels of virus too low to be detected (the last occurs only rarely when sensitive PCR or TMA assays are used). If the immunoblot test for anti-HCV is positive, the patient has most likely recovered from hepatitis C and has persistent antibody. If the immunoblot test is negative, the EIA result was probably a false positive.

Immunoblot tests are routine in blood banks when an anti-HCV-positive sample is found by EIA. Immunoblot assays are highly specific and valuable in verifying anti-HCV reactivity. Indeterminate tests require further followup testing, including attempts to confirm the specificity by repeat testing for HCV RNA.

Direct Assays for HCV RNA – PCR and TMA amplification can detect low levels of HCV RNA in serum. Testing for HCV RNA is a reliable way of demonstrating that hepatitis C infection is present and is the most specific test for infection. Testing for HCV RNA is particularly useful when aminotransferases are normal or only slightly elevated, when anti-HCV is not present, or when several causes of liver disease are possible. This method also helps diagnose hepatitis C in people who are immunosuppressed, have recently had an organ transplant, or have chronic renal failure. A PCR assay has now been approved by the Food and Drug Administration for general use. This assay will detect HCV RNA in serum down to a lower limit of 50 to 100 copies per milliliter (mL) which is equivalent to 25 to 50 international units (IU). A slightly more sensitive TMA test is currently under evaluation and may soon become available. Almost all patients with chronic hepatitis C will test positive by these assays.

Quantification of HCV RNA in Serum – Several methods are available for measuring the concentration or level of virus in serum, which is an indirect assessment of viral load. These methods include a quantitative PCR and a branched DNA (bDNA) test. Unfortunately, these assays are not well standardized, and different methods from different laboratories can provide different results on the same specimen. In addition, serum levels of HCV RNA can vary spontaneously by 3- to 10-fold over time. Nevertheless, when performed carefully, quantitative assays provide important insights into the nature of hepatitis C. Most patients with chronic hepatitis C have levels of HCV RNA (viral load) between 100,000 and 10,000,000 copies per mL. Expressed as IU, these averages are 50,000 to 5 million IU.

Viral levels as measured by HCV RNA do not correlate with the severity of the hepatitis or with a poor prognosis (as in HIV infection); but viral load does correlate with the likelihood of a response to antiviral therapy. Rates of response to a course of alpha interferon and ribavirin are higher in patients with low levels of HCV RNA. There are several definitions of a "low level" of HCV RNA, but the usual definition is below 1 million IU (2 million copies) per mL.

In addition, monitoring HCV RNA levels during the early phases of treatment may provide early information on the likelihood of a response. Yet because of the shortcomings of the current assays for HCV RNA level, these tests are not always reliable guides to therapy.

Genotyping and Serotyping of HCV – There are 6 known genotypes and more than 50 subtypes of hepatitis C. The genotype of infection is helpful in defining the epidemiology of hepatitis C. More important, knowing the genotype or serotype (genotype-specific antibodies) of HCV is helpful in making recommendations and counseling regarding therapy. Patients with genotypes 2 and 3 are two to three times more likely to respond to interferon-based therapy than patients with genotype 1.

Furthermore, when using combination therapy, the recommended dose and duration of treatment depend on the genotype. For patients with genotypes 2 and 3, a 24-week course of combination treatment using interferon and 800 milligrams (mg) of ribavirin daily is adequate, whereas for patients with genotype 1, a 48-week course and full dose of ribavirin (1,000 to 1,200 mg daily) is recommended. For these reasons, testing for HCV genotype is often clinically helpful. Once the genotype is identified, it need not be tested again; genotypes do not change during the course of infection.

> **Hepatitis D** – encapsulated by the hepatitis B surface antigen; without this coating, HDV cannot survive; must also, then, be the presence of HBV infection; hepatitis D is detected by the presence of **hepatitis D antigen (HDAg)** early on and **anti-HDV antibody (anti-HDV)** later. Both IgM and IgG **anti-HDV** arise later and persist indefinitely. The presence of **HDV RNA** confirms infection, but is only available in research laboratories.

- **Hepatitis D antigen (HDAg)** – rises early in the course of disease; indicates <u>acute infection</u>; also present in the <u>carrier state</u>..

- **Anti-HDV antibody (anti-HDV)** – appears later on; indicates <u>infectivity and chronic disease</u>.

Antibody/Antigen	Clinical Utility
HDAg	<ul><li>Generally disappears as HBsAg disappears</li><li>Most patients do not develop chronic infection</li><li>Only available in research laboratories</li></ul>
IgM anti-HDV	<ul><li>Present in most persons with with HBV-HDV co-infection</li><li>In 15%, detectable alone (without IgG anti-HDV) early in illness</li><li>Declines to sub-detectable levels after the infection resolves</li><li>No serologic marker persists to indicate that the patient was ever infected with HDV</li><li>Only available in research laboratories</li></ul>
IgG anti-HDV	<ul><li>Present in most persons with with HBV-HDV co-infection</li><li>In 15%, detectable alone (without IgM anti-HDV) during convalescence</li><li>Declines to sub-detectable levels after the infection resolves</li><li>No serologic marker that persists to indicate that the patient was ever infected with HDV</li><li>Test commercially available in the United States</li></ul>
HDV RNA	<ul><li>Confirms infection</li><li>Only available in research laboratories</li></ul>

In patients with chronic HBV infection who are super-infected with HDV several characteristic serologic features generally occur, including: 1) the titer of HBsAg declines at the time HDAg appears in the serum, 2) HDAg and HDV RNA remain detectable in the serum because chronic HDV infection generally occurs in most patients with HDV superinfection, unlike the case with co-infection, 3) high titers of both IgM and IgG anti-HDV are detectable, which persist indefinitely.

- **Hepatitis E** – a serologically distinct form of hepatitis that is rare in the US; no specific markers are commonly tested for here.

  All of the known serologic tests for HEV are only available in research laboratories.

Antibody	Clinical Utility
anti-HEV IgG	• May indicate past infection • May provide short term protection against the disease • False positive results are frequent • Only available in research laboratories
anti-HEV IgM	• Generally present during acute hepatitis E\ • Only available in research laboratories
HEV RNA	• Confirms diagnosis • Only available in research laboratories

- **Hepatitis F** – In 1994 an investigator reported finding viral particles in the stool of post-transfusion, non-A, non-B, non-C, non-E hepatitis cases. Injection of these particles to Indian rhesus monkeys presumably caused hepatitis, and they were named hepatitis F. Seven years later, another group suggested that these particles were actually a mutant form of HBV, rather than an entirely new virus. Subsequently, a group from New Delhi reported that the viral particles represented a"novel agent" that they called HFV. Separating "fact from fiction" in this ongoing debate is difficult. Currently, most clinicians do not recognize the existence of any form of hepatitis F.[2]

- **Hepatitis G** *(enrichment)* – Hepatitis G is a newly discovered form of liver inflammation caused by hepatitis G virus (HGV), a distant relative of the hepatitis C virus.

  Transfused blood containing HGV has caused some cases of hepatitis. HGV has been identified in between 1–2% of blood donors in the United States. Also at risk are patients with kidney disease who have blood exchange by hemodialysis, and those who inject drugs into their veins. It is possible that an infected mother can pass on the virus to her newborn infant. Sexual transmission also is a possibility.

  When diagnosed, acute HGV infection has usually been mild and brief. There is no evidence of serious complications, but it is possible that, like other hepatitis viruses, HGV can cause severe liver damage resulting in liver failure. The virus has been identified in as many as 20% of patients with long-lasting viral hepatitis, some of whom also have hepatitis C.

Diagnostic tests are not yet clinically available, but have been proven in research settings. During acute or chronic HGV infection, the only marker of that infection is the detection of viral RNA by polymerase chain reaction (PCR) assay or another molecular amplification technique. The presence of viral RNA is an accurate index of viremia and transmissibility.

Antibody to the envelope protein, E2, can be easily detected and appears to be an excellent marker of recovery from HGV infection and a powerful epidemiologic tool.[3] After the clearance of HGV RNA, antibody to the E2 envelope protein can be measured. Aside from a brief overlap period during recovery, HGV RNA and anti-E2 antibody are mutually exclusive, the former indicating ongoing viremia and the latter recovery from prior infection.[4]

No specific treatment is available for acute HGV infection. Since hepatitis G is a blood-borne infection, prevention relies on avoiding any possible contact with contaminated blood. Drug users should not share needles, syringes, or other equipment.

AIDS tests – used to diagnose the presence of the human immunodeficiency virus 1 and 2 in the blood. HIV-1 is more common in the US, while HIV-2 is more common in West Africa. The presence of the virus by itself does NOT necessarily indicate the presence of acquired immunodeficiency syndrome (AIDS). The diagnosis of AIDS requires confirmatory clinical and laboratory findings as well as a positive test for HIV.

- **Parameters measured:**   HIV antibody, CD4$^+$ lymphocyte levels, CD8$^+$ lymphocyte levels, plasma HIV RNA (viral load), HIV drug resistance testing

- **The test in a "nutshell":**   Determines, along with clinical features, the presence of HIV infection and the diagnosis of AIDS (HIV antibody tests). Allows the clinician to identify the immunocompetence and prognosis of the affected patient, as well as the response to therapy (CD4$^+$ lymphocyte levels, CD8$^+$ lymphocyte levels, plasma HIV RNA [viral load], HIV drug resistance testing).

- **Normal values:**

Parameter	Normal value (adults)
HIV antibody	Negative
CD4$^+$ lymphocyte levels	600-1500 cells/mm^3
CD8$^+$ lymphocyte levels	300-800 cells/mm^3
Plasma HIV RNA (viral load)	No viral RNA detected
HIV drug resistance testing	No resistance noted

PANIC VALUES!!

CD4$^+$ lymphocytes < 500
Viral load > 100,000 copies/ml

- **Results in a "nutshell":**

PARAMETER	IMPLICATIONS
HIV antibody	Confirmed positive value usually diagnostic of HIV infection; clinical picture required to determine whether or not AIDS is also present. Also helpful for screening prior to use in transfusion.
CD4$^+$ lymphocyte levels	Determines degree of immunocompetence of host; decreases indicate need (at specific levels) for prophylactic treatment of opportunistic infections (e.g., *pneumocystis carinii*).
CD8$^+$ lymphocyte levels	Indicate degree of immunocompetence of host; exact role in HIV infection and AIDS is not completely clear.
Plasma HIV RNA (viral load)	Indicates the level of HIV activity in the body. Combined with CD4$^+$ levels and clinical features, helps determine when to start antiretroviral therapy.
HIV drug resistance testing	Helps determine if the virus is susceptible to a particular therapeutic agent; useful when treatment failure or reversion of previously successful therapy occurs.

■ **Test Details**

1. Diagnostic antibody tests – HIV antibodies generally do not reach detectable levels in the blood for one to three months following infection. It may take the antibodies as long as six months to be produced in quantities large enough to show up in standard blood tests.

    People exposed to the virus should get an HIV test as soon as they are likely to develop antibodies to the virus – within 6 weeks to 12 months after possible exposure to the virus. By getting tested early, people with HIV infection can discuss with a health care provider when they should start treatment to help their immune systems combat HIV and help prevent the emergence of certain opportunistic infections. Early testing also alerts HIV-infected people to avoid high-risk behaviors that could spread the virus to others.

    - **HIV Antibody (HTLV-III antibody)** – used to diagnose AIDS and to screen blood for use in transfusion. The test detects HIV antibody by an enzyme-linked immunosorbent assay (ELISA) and a positive test is usually confirmed by the Western blot test.

    - **Western Blot Analysis for AIDS** – the technique used as the reference procedure for confirming the presence or absence of HIV antibody, usually after a positive HIV antibody by ELISA determination. The HIV antigen is purified using gel electrophoresis, then attached to a nitrocellulose filter against which the serum suspected of antibody positivity is reacted; an enzyme labeled antihuman immunoglobulin is reacted with the complex followed by a chromogenic substrate to visualize the reaction.

2. Lymphocyte subsets – T cells are involved in cell-mediated immunity. Two types of T cells are $CD4^+$ (helper) and $CD8^+$ (suppressor or cytotoxic) cells. HIV causes a slow decline in $CD4^+$ cells in most people. Normal $CD4^+$ cell counts are 600–1,500 cells per cubic millimeter of blood. Normal $CD8^+$ cell counts in an HIV-negative person are 300–800 cells per cubic millimeter of blood.

    According to the most recently published guidelines,[5] the $CD4^+$ T-cell count (or CD4 count) serves as the major clinical indicator of immunocompetence in patients with HIV infection. It is usually the most important consideration in decisions to initiate antiretroviral therapy. The most recent CD4 cell count is the strongest predictor of subsequent disease progression and survival, according to clinical trials and cohort studies data on patients receiving antiretroviral therapy.

    - Use of CD4 for initial assessment – the CD4 count is usually the most important consideration in decisions to initiate antiretroviral therapy. All patients should have a baseline CD4 cell count at entry into care.

- Use of CD4 count for monitoring therapeutic response – adequate viral suppression for most patients on therapy is defined as an increase in CD4 cell count that averages 100-150 cells/mm^3 per year with an accelerated response in the first three months. This is largely due to redistribution. Subsequent increases with good virologic control show an average increase of approximately 100 cells/mm^3 per year for the subsequent few years until a threshold is reached.[6]

- Frequency of CD4 count monitoring – in general, the CD4 count should be determined every three to four months to (1) determine when to start antiretroviral in patients who do not meet the criteria for initiation; (2) assess immunologic response to antiretroviral therapy; and (3) assess the need for initating chemoprophylaxis for opportunistic infections.

CD4$^+$ cell counts, not viral load, are a better indicator for when to start preventive therapy for opportunistic infections. The significance of different CD4$^+$ counts is summarized in the table below:

CD4$^+$ CELL COUNT	ASSOCIATED RISKS
Above 500 CD4$^+$ cells	No unusual conditions likely
200–500 CD4$^+$ cells	Increased risk for shingles (zoster), thrush (candida), skin infections, bacterial, sinus, lung infections, and TB. Opportunistic infections (such as pneumocystis [PCP], mycobacterium avium complex (MAC), or cytomegalovirus [CMV] are rare.
50–200 CD4$^+$ cells	Increased risk for PCP and other opportunistic infections. Preventative treatment for PCP (e.g., sulfamethoxazole-trimethoprim [Septra®] is indicated. Consider prophylaxis for MAC and CMV.
Below 50 CD4$^+$ cells	Increased risk for opportunistic infections, including MAC and CMV; prophylaxis recommended

Some use the CD4$^+$ percentage (normal = 28-58%) of total lymphocytes or the CD4+/CD8$^+$ ratio (normally ~ 2), to monitor disease progression.

3. Viral load – viral load (also known as plasma HIV RNA) measures the actual amount of viral RNA present in the body. This is an excellent indication of the stage of a patient's disease and it's progression. Viral load is also used to monitor response to therapy. Newer testing methods are extremely sensitive and are accurate in sensing as few as 50 copies of viral RNA. Using both

$CD4^+$ counts and viral load testing provides a more complete picture of a person's risk of disease progression and response to therapy. While $CD4^+$ cell counts indicate the status of a person's immune system, viral load tests indicate the activity of the virus.

Combined with $CD4^+$ counts, viral load is also helpful in monitoring persons who are HIV positive, but have not yet developed full-blown clinical AIDS. Higher viral load correlates with lower $CD4^+$ counts, more rapid declines in $CD4^+$ cell counts and more rapid disease progression. People with viral load levels over 100,000 copies/ml have been shown to be ten times more likely to progress to AIDS over the following five years compared to those with levels below 100,000 copies/ml . People with constant viral load levels below 10,000 copies/ml seem to have a lowered risk of disease progression.[7]

The general interpretation of viral loads is as follows:

- Low = less than 10,000 copies/ml
- High = greater than 100,000 copies/ml

Low, stable, or decreasing viral load is considered good. High or increasing levels are worrisome, as they may indicate treatment failure.

Since viral loads often deal with very large numbers, they are sometimes expressed in terms of logarithms. This is a mathematical scale (remember the days of algebra?) that "compresses" large numbers into simpler ones. The details will not be reviewed here. The minimum reliable change in measurements is a 3-fold (0.5 log) change (this means 3 times larger or smaller than the last test result). Thus a change from 20,000 down to 10,000 (a 2-fold change) would not be considered reliable and significant (although repeated tests showing the same change would validate the result). Any lower decrease may only be due to testing errors, other infections or normal biological fluctuations.

Three HIV viral load assays have been approved by the Food and Drug Administration (FDA) for clinical use:[8]

- HIV-1 reverse transcriptase polymerase chain reaction assay (Amplicor HIV-1 Monitor Test®, version 1.5, Roche Diagnostic)
- Nucleic acid amplification test for HIV RNA (NucliSens HIV-1 QT®, Organon Teknika)
- Signal amplification nucleic acid probe assay (VERSANT HIV-1RNA 3.0 assay®, Bayer).

Analysis of 18 trials with over 5,000 participants with viral load monitoring showed a significant association between a decrease in plasma viremia and improved clinical outcome. Thus, viral load testing serves as a surrogate marker for treatment response and may be useful in predicting clinical progression. The minimal change in viral load considered to be statistically significant (2 standard deviations) is a threefold or a 0.5 log10 copies/mL change. One key goal of therapy is a viral load below the limits of detection (at <50 copies/mL for the Amplicor® assay, <75 copies/mL for the VERSANT® assay, and <80 copies/mL for the NucliSens® assay). This goal should be achieved by 16-24 weeks. Recommendations for monitoring of the viral load are as follows:

- At initiation or change in therapy – plasma viral load should be measured immediately before treatment, and at 2-8 weeks after treatment initiation or treatment changes due to suboptimal viral suppression.

- In patients with viral suppression where changes are motivated by drug toxicity or regimen simplification – some experts also recommend repeating viral load measurement within 2-8 weeks after changing therapy. The purpose of viral load monitoring at this point is to confirm potency of the new regimen.

- In patients on a stable antiretroviral regimen – the viral load testing should be repeated every 3-4 months thereafter or if clinically indicated.

4. When to start antiretroviral treatment – for previously untreated patients the newest recommendations, cited above, use a combination of the $CD4^+$ count and viral load to estimate the risk of disease-free survival. The Panel's recommendations are as follows:[9]

- Antiretroviral therapy is recommended for all patients with history of an AIDS-defining illness or severe symptoms of HIV infection regardless of $CD4^+$ T cell count.
- Antiretroviral therapy is also recommended for asymptomatic patients with <200 $CD4^+$ T cells/mm^3
- Asymptomatic patients with $CD4^+$ T cell counts of 201-350 cells/mm^3 should be offered treatment.
- For asymptomatic patients with $CD4^+$ T cell of >350 cells/mm^3 and plasma HIV RNA >100,000 copies/ml most experienced clinicians defer therapy but some clinicians may consider initiating treatment.
- Therapy should be deferred for patients with $CD4^+$ T cell counts of >350 cells /mm^3 and plasma HIV RNA <100,000 copies/mL.

5. Drug resistance testing – the Panel made the following recommendations regarding drug resistance testing:

- HIV drug resistance testing should be performed to assist in selecting active drugs when changing antiretroviral regimens in cases of virologic failure.
- Drug resistance testing should also be considered when managing suboptimal viral load reduction.

- Drug resistance testing in the setting of virologic failure should be performed while the patient is taking antiretroviral drugs, or immediately (i.e, within 4 weeks) after discontinuing therapy.
- If the decision is made to initiate therapy in a person with acute HIV infection, it is likely that resistance testing at baseline will optimize virologic response; this strategy should b considered.
- Drug resistance testing at baseline in antiretroviral-naïve, chronically infected patients i an untested strategy. However, it may be reasonable to consider resistance testing when there is a significant probability that the patient was infected with a drug-resistance viru i.e., if the patient is thought to have been infected by a person who was receiving antiretroviral drugs.
- Drug resistance testing is not advised for persons with viral load <1,000 copies/mL, sin amplification of the virus is unreliable.

There are two types of resistance assays for use in assessing viral strains and selecting treatmen strategies: genotypic and phenotypic assays.

- Genotypic assays – genotyping assays detect drug resistance mutations that are present the relevant viral genes. Certain genotyping assays involve sequencing of the entire reverse transcriptase and protease genes, whereas others use probes to detect selected mutations that are known to confer drug resistance. Genotypic assays can be performed rapidly, and results can be reported within 1-2 weeks of sample collection. Interpretatio of test results requires knowledge of the mutations that are selected for by different antiretroviral drugs and of the potential for cross-resistance to other drugs conferred by certain mutations.

- Phenotypic assays – phenotyping assays measure a virus's ability to grow in different concentrations of antiretroviral drugs. Automated phenotyping assays are commercially available with results available in 2-3 weeks. However, phenotyping assays are more costly to perform than genotyping assays. Drug concentrations that inhibit 50% and 90% of viral replication are calculated. Interpretation of phenotyping assay results is complicated by the paucity of data regarding the specific resistance level that is associated with drug failure, although clinically significant fold increase cutoffs are now available for some drugs.

Consultation with a specialist in HIV drug resistance can help clinicians best utilize the above tests. Further limitations of both genotyping and phenotyping assays include the lack of uniforr quality assurance for all available assays, relatively high cost, and insensitivity for minor viral species. If drug-resistant viruses are present but constitute <10%-20% of the circulating virus population, they probably will not be detected by available assays. No definitive prospective data exist to support using one type of resistance assay over another (i.e., genotyping versus phenotyping) in different clinical situations. Therefore, one type of assay is recommended per sample.

6.   Lab tests and assessment of antiretroviral treatment failure – Antiretroviral treatment failure can be defined as a suboptimal response to therapy. Any of a number of factors may be the cause, including regimen complexity that hinders adherence, medication intolerance and toxicity, suboptimal pharmacokinetics, inadequate antiviral potency, drug resistance, etc. Treatment failure is often associated with virologic failure, immunologic failure, and/or clinical progression:

- Virologic failure – can be defined as incomplete or lack of HIV RNA response to antiretroviral therapy:

   ▸ Incomplete virologic response – this can be defined as repeated HIV RNA >400 copies/mL after 24 weeks or >50 copies/mL by 48 weeks in a treatment-naïve patient initiating therapy. Baseline HIV RNA may impact the time course of response and some patients will take longer than others to suppress HIV RNA levels. The timing, pattern, and/or slope of HIV RNA decrease may predict the ultimate virologic response.

   ▸ Virologic rebound – after virologic suppression, repeated detection of HIV RNA.

- Immunologic failure can be defined as failure to increase the CD4 cell count by 25-50 cells/mm^3 above the baseline count over the first year of therapy, or a decrease to below the baseline CD4 cell count on therapy. Mean increases in CD4 cell counts in treatment-naïve patients with initial antiretroviral regimens are approximately 150 cells/mm^3 over the first year.[10] A lower baseline CD4 cell count may be associated with less of a response to therapy. For reasons not fully understood, some patients may have initial CD4 cell increases, but then minimal subsequent increases. Immunologic failure (i.e., return to baseline CD4 cell count) occurred an average of 3 years following virologic failure in patients remaining on the same antiretroviral regimen.[11]

- Clinical progression can be defined as the occurrence or recurrence of HIV-related events (after at least 3 months on an antiretroviral regimen), excluding immune reconstitution syndromes.[12] In one study, clinical progression (a new AIDS event or death) occurred in 7% of treated patients with virologic suppression, 9% of treated patients with virologic rebound, and 20% of treated patients who never achieved virologic suppression over 2.5 years.[13]

Relationship across virologic failure, immunologic failure, and clinical progression. Some patients demonstrate discordant responses in virologic, immunologic and clinical parameters.[14] In addition, virologic failure, immunologic failure, and clinical progression have distinct time courses and may occur independently or simultaneously. In general, virologic failure occurs first, followed by immunologic failure, and finally by clinical progression. These events may be separated by months to years.

CHAPTER 7 – ARTERIAL BLOOD GASES
PARAMETERS MEASURED
THE TEST IN A "NUTSHELL"
NORMAL VALUES
PANIC VALUES
RESULTS IN A "NUTSHELL"
TEST DETAILS
ARTERIAL BLOOD GASES MADE SIMPLE

CHAPTER 7 – ARTERIAL BLOOD GASES

Arterial blood gases (ABGs) are a common test that provides the clinician with useful and potentially life-saving therapy. The discussion below will discuss only the parameters that are actually measured on the ABG, *not* the calculated numbers (e.g., base excess, bicarbonate). It is the author's (and many other of our colleague's) opinion that these calculated parameters do not help in our clinical care of the patient and only serve to confuse us.

- **Parameters measured:**   pH, pCO_2, pO_2

- **The test in a "nutshell":**   Assesses adequacy of oxygenation (pO_2), ventilation (pH, pCO_2), and acid-base balance (pH, pCO_2). Commonly ordered to evaluate acid-base balance, shortness of breath.

- **Normal values (room air, sea level):**

pH	7.35-7.45
pCO_2	35-45 mmHg (torr)
pO_2	> 80 mmHg (torr)

PANIC VALUES!!

pH < 7.25 or > 7.55
pCO_2 > 60 mmHg
pO_2 < 50 mmHg

- **Results in a "nutshell":**

PARAMETER	IMPLICATIONS
pH	Measures degree of acidity or alkalinity in the arterial blood; elevated values indicate **alkalosis**, decreased values indicate **acidosis**.
pCO_2	The **partial pressure** of carbon dioxide in the arterial blood; modulated by the respiratory system; an index of **ventilation**.
pO_2	Partial pressure of oxygen in arterial blood; low values indicate **hypoxia**; should increase in response to supplemental oxygen.

■   **Test details**

pH

▸   The **pH** measures the acidity or alkalinity of the blood. The $[H^+]$ is directly proportiona[l]
to the acidity or alkalinity of the blood (high $[H^{+]}$ = acidotic; lower $[H^+]$ = alkalotic).
Mathematically, pH is defined as the **negative logarithm of the hydrogen ion
concentration**:

pH = -Logarithm (Base 10) of the concentration of H^+

▸   More important than the mathematics is the fact that the pH scale is a **logarithmic** one.
A change of 1 pH unit represents a 10-**fold** change in the $[H^+]$, a change of 2, a 100-**fold**
change, etc.

▸   The normal pH of arterial blood is 7.40. An acceptable range is usually defined as 7.35-
7.45. Values above this indicate the presence of a basic (**alkalotic**) state. Values below
suggest an acidic content to the blood (**acidosis**).

▸   Technically, an alkalosis or acidosis refers to a *process* that results in the presence of
either an **alkalemia** or an **acidemia**. This is a moot semantic point. For purposes of our
discussion, we will use the terms interchangeably. Thus the arterial blood pH indicates
whether the blood is acidotic, alkalotic, or normal in terms of acid-base balance. This is
illustrated in the examples below:

pH = 7.56 — too high → alkalosis
pH = 7.23 — too low → acidosis
pH = 7.38 — just right → normal

pCO$_2$

▸   The pCO$_2$ represents the **partial pressure of carbon dioxide** in arterial blood. The unit[s]
are the same as those for pO$_2$. The normal value (at all altitudes) averages 40 mm Hg.
An acceptable range is 35-42 or so. As the pCO$_2$ increases, so does the acidity of the
blood (i.e., the pH will decrease).

▸   As the pCO$_2$ decreases, the alkalinity (and pH) will *increase*. Changes in the pCO$_2$ are
effected by respiration. Hyperventilation will "blow off" more CO$_2$, leading to a
decreased pCO$_2$, thus an increased pH. In cases of respiratory failure, CO$_2$ is not "blow[n]
off" properly. It accumulates in the blood, leading to an increased pCO$_2$ and a decrease[d]
the pH.

▸   High or low pCO_2 levels may be a *primary* response to a respiratory condition or a *secondary* response to some other problem elsewhere in the body. Usually, a secondary response occurs when a metabolic condition has changed the pH significantly. The body attempts to compensate by changing respiration to either increase or decrease the excretion of CO_2. This occurs relatively rapidly. When a primary respiratory problem changes the pCO_2 and, thus, the pH, the body also tries to compensate metabolically. This process takes a while longer and will not be discussed here.

pO_2

▸   The pO_2 represents the **partial pressure of oxygen** in the arterial blood. It is measured in millimeters of mercury (mm Hg). The normal pO_2 depends on the altitude. Generally, breathing room air, the sea level pO_2 should be 80-100 mm Hg. Values considerably lower than this indicate room air **hypoxia**.

▸   The pO_2 should, of course, increase with the presence of supplemental O_2.

Classification of acid-base disorders

▸   We can define acid-base deviations as either **alkalosis** (basic, pH > 7.45) or **acidosis** (acid, pH < 7.35).

▸   Either condition can be caused by respiratory or metabolic problems.

▸   Depending on the time involved, either primary problem may be *partially compensated for* by a secondary process. This is not always the case, though.

1.   **Respiratory acidosis and alkalosis**

▸   **Pure respiratory acidosis** involves the retention (usually acutely) of CO_2 due to either hypoventilation (i.e., drug overdose) or intrinsic lung disease (COPD, ARDS). The pCO_2 is increased (> 45) and the pH is decreased below 7.35. The pO_2 is usually decreased but this value is irrelevant in diagnosing the acid-base state. It should be viewed *separately!*

▸   A **pure respiratory alkalosis** involves "blowing off" CO_2, usually due to hyperventilation (for any of a number of causes). The pCO_2 is decreased (below 35) and the pH increased above 7.45.

▸   Examples of ABGs demonstrating these conditions are shown below:

Case 1 — 21-year-old male with acute respiratory failure from narcotic intoxication. Respiratory rate = 4/minute. pH = 7.2O, pCO_2 = 60, pO_2 = 45. This patient is retaining CO_2 due to hypoventilation. The pH is *decreased,* indicating an acidosis. The pCO_2 is *increased,* indicating a respiratory acidosis.

Case 2 — 35-year-old female with pleuritic chest pain and a pulmonary embolism. Her respiratory rate is 35/min. pH = 7.60, pCO_2 = 20, pO_2 = 55. This patient is hyperventilating, thus "blowing off CO_2. This lowers her pCO_2 and increases the blood pH. The increased pH indicates an alkalosis. The decreased pCO_2 defines a **respiratory alkalosis.**

2.   **Metabolic acidosis and alkalosis**

▸   **A pure metabolic acidosis** involves the abnormal production and/or retention of metabolic acids or loss of base. The pH is *decreased,* indicating a higher hydrogen ion concentration (the H^+ concentration is directly proportional to the acidity of the blood). The pCO_2, at least initially, is unchanged.

▸   A **pure metabolic alkalosis** occurs with loss of acid or massive increase in metabolic base. The pH is *increased* indicating a lower H^+ ion concentration. Again, initially, the pCO_2 is unchanged.

▸   Examples of these processes are shown below:

Case 3 — 60-year-old male who goes into acute renal failure following an intravenous pyelogram. pH = 7.25, pCO_2 = 37, pO_2 = 70. The pH is decreased, indicating an **acidosis.** The PCO_2 is normal. This indicates that there is NO respiratory component. This indicates the patient has a **pure metabolic acidosis**

Case 4—a 45-year-old woman who has received NG suction for the last 36 hour and inappropriate fluid-replacement. (NG suction removes stomach acid and commonly leads to an alkalotic state.) pH = 7.56, pCO_2 = 35, pO_2 = 80. The pH *increased,* indicating an **alkalosis.** The pCO_2 *is normal,* meaning, again, there is NO respiratory component. Thus, the patient has a **pure metabolic alkalosis.**

Mixed acid-base disturbances

Rather than try to remember complex rules and formulas to decide whether an acid-base disturbance is "pure" or "mixed," try the following:

1.   ***Look at the pH***. Is it high, low, or normal? A high pH defines an *alkalosis;* a low pH defines an *acidosis.* A normal pH may mean no acid-base disturbance or the result of tw or more disturbances which "balance each other out."

2. ***Look at the pCO_2.*** If it is elevated, there is a component of respiratory acidosis. An *elevated pCO_2* with a *decreased pH* = **pure respiratory acidosis.** An *elevated PCO_2 with a normal* or *increased pH* = primary metabolic process *(alkalosis)* with a **compensatory respiratory acidosis.** If the pCO_2 is decreased, there is a component of respiratory alkalosis present. A *decreased pCO_2* with an *increased pH* = **pure respiratory alkalosis.** A *decreased pCO_2* with a *normal* or *decreased pH* = primary metabolic process (acidosis) with a compensatory respiratory alkalosis.

    In other words, the pCO_2 and pH should deviate in *opposite directions* in primary respiratory processes and in the *same direction* in compensatory respiratory processes. If the pCO_2 is normal, the acidosis/alkalosis is a primary metabolic problem with no significant attempt at respiratory compensation.

3. ***Look at the pO_2.*** *You* should also determine, in addition to acid-base status, if the patient is hypoxemic or not. pO_2 is a measurement of **oxygenation**, not of ventilation.

General approach to ABGs

▶   All you really need to know is the following:

1. Is the patient acidotic/alkalotic?
2. If so, is it *primarily* a respiratory or a metabolic process?
3. Is the patient hypoxemic?

In summary:

▶   **If by pH there is an acidosis and the pCO_2 is**:

Elevated – pure respiratory acidosis

Decreased – metabolic acidosis with respiratory compensation

Normal – metabolic acidosis without respiratory compensation

▶   **If by pH there is an alkalosis and the pCO_2 is**:

Decreased – pure respiratory alkalosis

Elevated – metabolic alkalosis with respiratory compensation

Normal – metabolic alkalosis without respiratory compensation

Condition	pH	pCO$_2$
Pure respiratory alkalosis	High	Low
Pure respiratory acidosis	Low	High
Pure metabolic alkalosis	High	Normal
Pure metabolic acidosis	Low	Normal
Metabolic alkalosis with respiratory compensation	High	High
Metabolic acidosis with respiratory compensation	Low	Low

Additional case examples

Case 5 – 35-year-old female with diabetic ketoacidosis. Her respiratory rate is 25. pH = 7.25, pCO$_2$ = 20, pO$_2$ = 110. The pH is low indicating an acidosis. The pCO$_2$ is also low. Thus, there is also a **respiratory alkalosis.** This suggests a **metabolic acidosis** (lowering the pH) with a **compensatory respiratory alkalosis** (hyperventilating in an attempt to correct the metabolic acidosis by creating a respiratory alkalosis). This is a commonly observed pattern in diabetic ketoacidosis.

Case 6 – 20-year-old male with an acute asthma attack. Despite three nebulized albuterol treatments, he's still very "tight" and short of breath. His respiratory rate is 40. pH = 7.30, pCO$_2$ = 50, pO$_2$ = 59. The pH is low indicating an **acidosis.** The pCO$_2$ *is elevated.* Thus, this patient has a **respiratory acidosis.** There is also significant hypoxemia.

Case 7 – 65-year-old male with a "cold." He is coughing up copious amounts of greenish sputum. There is a known history of COPD. Patient's respiratory rate = 35/min, pH = 7.35, pCO$_2$ = 70. PO$_2$ = 50. (This is somewhat of a "trick" question but highly relevant). The pH is *normal* (a bit toward the low side). The pCO$_2$ is *elevated.* This suggests a **respiratory acidosis**, but why is the pH normal? The reason is because this patient is a chronic CO$_2$ retainer. His body has become used to this condition and fought it by developing a **chronic metabolic alkalosis**. If you measured the patient's serum bicarbonate level, it would be markedly elevated, proving the hypothesis. Thus, this gentleman has a **primary respiratory acidosis** with a **compensatory metabolic alkalosis.**

Case 8 – the same patient as in *case 7*, except that he appears to be more obtunded. ABGs now show pH = 7.15, pCO$_2$ = 110, and pO$_2$ = 75. There is now a significant **acidosis.** The pCO$_2$ is *markedly elevated* indicating a severe **respiratory acidosis.** Thus, there is an **acute respiratory acidosis** superimposed upon a **chronic respiratory acidosis** with a **compensatory metabolic alkalosis.** This is exactly the type of acid-base pattern a chronic CO$_2$ retainer will develop when they acutely decompensate.

104

ARTERIAL BLOOD GASES MADE SIMPLE (REALLY!) *[enrichment]*[15]

More health care professionals lose sleep over arterial blood gases (ABGs) than just about any other lab test we get. I just can't believe how complex this straightforward test is made to appear. *PLEASE* — try it my way; thousands of our colleagues who had near panic attacks in the past are now very comfortable with ABGs.

> **REMEMBER**: ABGs *are* easy and straight-forward. Unfortunately, few of us were lucky enough to learn these facts the first time around!

You only need to look at four items — and *one* of them is the patient's name. The other three are: pH, pCO_2, and pO_2. Just about everything else on an ABG report represents calculated parameters that are *not needed* to identify the primary underlying acid-base disorder in most patients. Try it — I guarantee results ☺ . . .

NORMAL ABG VALUES (SEA LEVEL)

pH	**7.35-7.45**
pCO_2	**35-45 mm Hg (torr)**
pO_2	**> 80 mm Hg (torr)**

NOTE: torr is another unit of pressure that is sometimes used interchangeably with mm Hg

Why we get confused reading ABGs. There are three main reasons we have trouble with ABGs:

1. *Trying to figure out all the extraneous material on the report* — thus, my suggestion is to look at only the four most important items — the patient's name, pH, pCO_2, and pO_2.

2. *Trying to make pH, pCO_2, and pO_2 interrelate predictably.* It just doesn't happen that way (remember why the apple fell on Newton's head — don't try to rock the boat and rewrite the laws of physics!). True, there is a solid "marriage" between pH and pCO_2, which we'll talk about shortly. However, the relationship between pCO_2 and pO_2 is far less predictable. One day, they get along; the next, you find yourself in the middle of an ugly "domestic" situation. Get the hint?

3. *Always trying to find a logical correlation between the pH and pCO_2 on the ABG and the serum bicarbonate level on the electrolyte panel.* Remember when I said that findings on the bicarbonate level were *independent* of the pH and pCO_2? At least for now, assume that the pH, pCO_2, and pO_2 are *independent* of the serum bicarbonate level on the electrolyte panel.

With the above *caveats* in mind, let's make sure we understand what each of the three measured parameters really means . . .

Separate and only sometimes-related physiological processes. The arterial pH, pCO_2, and pO_2 represent separate physiological processes. Sometimes, they are closely related; other times not:

- **pH** — represents acid-base balance; the sum of all respiratory and metabolic acid-base processes.

- **pCO_2** — chemically, the partial pressure of CO_2 dissolved in the blood. It is a respiratory acid, and is controlled by the lungs. The process of CO_2 exchange is known as **ventilation**. Changes in the pCO_2 result in near-instantaneous changes in the pH (unlike changes in the serum bicarbonate, which may take hours to days to occur, if at all).

- **pO_2** — chemically, the partial pressure of O_2 dissolved in the blood. The process of O_2 exchange is known as **oxygenation**.

What causes cyanosis? Cyanosis is not related directly to the pO_2. It appears whenever the arterial blood contains more than five grams of deoxygenated hemoglobin per 100 milliliters of blood. Anemic patients rarely show significant cyanosis because they don't have enough hemoglobin for five grams of it to be deoxygenated in the arterial blood. On the other hand, patients with polycythemia have excess available hemoglobin and may appear cyanotic, even under otherwise normal conditions.

The "happy marriage." Oxygenation and ventilation are not always directly related. On the other hand, ventilation (pCO_2) and acid-base balance (pH) *are* predictably related ("happily married forever"). Remember that respiratory changes occur rapidly through the lungs, versus metabolic ones, which take hours to days via the kidney:

- pCO_2 represents *respiratory acid*. **Increased** blood levels of pCO_2 means *increased* acid, therefore *decreased* pH.

- Since pCO_2 represents respiratory acid, **decreases** in the blood pCO_2 level mean a *decrease* in acid, therefore *increased* pH.

Do you notice a pattern? Sure hope so. With a *decrease* in the pCO_2 there is an *increase* in the pH, and vice versa. This "marriage" is so stable because of this predictable inverse relationship: *when the pCO_2 moves one way, the pH always moves in the* opposite *direction*. In fact, we can quantitate this relationship as follows: *for every 10 mg Hg increase or decrease in pCO_2, the pH moves 0.1 units in the* opposite *direction*. Make certain you are comfortable why this has to be true. Increased pCO_2 levels add acid (more acidotic), lowering the pH; decreased pCO_2 levels take away acid (more alkalotic), leading to an increase in the pH. The 10 to 0.1 ratio merely represents empiric findings — use it to your favor.

Now, let's put it all together using a simple, yet elegant, "three question approach."

I have only three questions — To properly identify the primary underlying abnormality (respiratory/metabolic, acidosis/alkalosis) follow these rules:

1.   Look at the pO_2. **Is it low?** If it's low, *fix it*! Otherwise, move on to the next step. I'm not trying to minimize the importance of hypoxia; once you've identified it, the presence contributes nothing more to the test interpretation. Give oxygen and look at the pH.

2.   Look at the pH. Assuming it's not normal, is it too high or too low? If it's normal, maybe the test shouldn't have been done in the first place — or there is a compensatory process present. Patients *rarely* completely compensate, at least acutely, and *never* overcompensate. For the sake of understanding, let's just learn the system with either a high pH (alkalotic) or a low pH (acidotic). Note that the suffix "tic" refers to the net pH, while "sis" refers to a *process*. There may be more than one process contributing to the net pH. Our system helps identify the *primary* culprit — yes, there is always an "instigator," regardless of what else might be going on. So, look at what the pH did — **which way did it go, up (too high; alkalotic) or down (too low; acidotic)?**

3.   Look at the pCO_2. Only one question left: **"Did the pCO_2 move in the *opposite* direction as the pH?"** If so, the primary underlying process is *respiratory*. If not, the primary underlying process is *metabolic*. Trust me on this one, and please understand why these statements are correct; don't just memorize (though the "cookbook approach" *is* correct as well as helpful). Note, I didn't ask the alternative two questions (did the pCO_2 move in the *same* direction as the pH or not change at all?). Why ask two questions when one will do?

        Think about it — if the pCO_2 and pH move in opposite directions, the primary process *must* be respiratory, based on the 10 to 0.1 ratio discussed above. Otherwise, the primary process *must* be metabolic, and the pCO_2 remains unchanged or moves in the *same* direction as the pH.

Combining the pH and pCO_2 information as above, it's simple to classify the primary process as either alkalosis or acidosis (depending on whether the pH is too high or too low), and either respiratory or metabolic (depending on whether the pCO_2 moves in the *opposite* direction of the pH). Don't try to make the process more complicated than it really is. If you follow this system, you're going to get it right most of the time!

Let's try some examples to be sure. For our purposes here (and to make my math easy), let's assume that the normal pH is 7.40, the pCO_2 is 40 mm Hg, and the pO_2 is greater than 80 mm Hg.

Example 1 — 21-year-old male with acute narcotic intoxication. His respiratory rate is 4/min.

Parameter	Patient	Normal
pH	7.20	7.35-7.45
pCO2	60	35-45 mm Hg (torr)
pO$_2$	45	> 80 mm Hg (torr)

Now, ask the "three questions":

1. Look at the pO$_2$. Is it low?. It's *too low*; the patient is hypoxic, so please fix it. Now, move on the next question.

2. Look at the pH. Assuming it's not normal, is it too high or too low? It's *too low*; thus, the patient is acidotic — the pH went *down*. Only one question left . . .

3. Look at the pCO$_2$. Did it move opposite from the pH? The pH went *down*, so we are really asking if the pCO$_2$ went *up*? Well, did it? You bet. Since the pH and pCO$_2$ moved in *opposite* directions, the primary underlying problem is *respiratory*.

Putting everything together, the patient has a *respiratory acidosis* with concomitant hypoxia. Of course, in light of the clinical history, it shouldn't surprise us that the pO$_2$ would be low, unless the patient overdoses in a hyperbaric chamber!

Now, lets *prove* that we're right, rather than memorizing. Here, let's simply ask what would the effect on pCO$_2$ *have* to be if, via a primary respiratory process, he (the overdosed male) retained 20 "units" of pCO$_2$? Based on our 10 to 0.1 "opposite" ratio above, an increase of 20 mm Hg in the pCO$_2$ should *decrease* the pH by 0.2 units — which is exactly what happened. Thus, we've proven that the system works so far. Let's try another case . . .

Example 2 — 35-year-old female with pleuritic chest pain; her respiratory rate is 35/min.

Parameter	Patient	Normal
pH	7.60	7.35-7.45
pCO2	20	35-45 mm Hg (torr)
pO$_2$	55	> 80 mm Hg (torr)

Now, ask the "three questions":

1.   Look at the pO$_2$. Is it low?. It's *too low*; the patient is hypoxic, so please fix it. Now, move on to the next question.

2.   Look at the pH. Assuming it's not normal, is it too high or too low? It's *too high;* thus, the patient is alkalotic — the pH went *up.* Only one question left . . .

3.   Look at the pCO$_2$. Did it move opposite from the pH? The pH went *up,* so we are really asking if the pCO$_2$ went *down.* Well, did it? You bet. Since the pH and pCO$_2$ moved in *opposite* directions, the primary underlying problem is *respiratory*.

Putting everything together, the patient has a *respiratory alkalosis* with concomitant hypoxia. The low pO$_2$ points out why we should always *assume* that even the most "obvious" anxiety-hyperventilator has something seriously wrong until proven otherwise.

Again, lets *prove* that we're right, rather than memorizing. Here, let's ask what would the effect on pCO$_2$ *have* to be if, via a primary respiratory process, we "blew off" 20 "units" of pCO$_2$? Based on our 10 to 0.1 "opposite" ratio above, a decrease of 20 mm Hg in the pCO$_2$ should *increase* the pH by 0.2 units — which is exactly what happened. Thus, we've proven that the system works, again. Here's your next patient:

Example 3 — 60-year-old male in acute renal failure following an intravenous pyelogram.

Parameter	Patient	Normal
pH	7.25	7.35-7.45
pCO2	40	35-45 mm Hg (torr)
pO$_2$	70	> 80 mm Hg (torr)

Now, ask the "three questions":

1.   Look at the pO$_2$. Is it low?. It's *too low*; the patient is hypoxic, so please fix it. Now, move on to the next question.

2.   Look at the pH. Assuming it's not normal, is it too high or too low? It's *too low*; thus, the patient is acidotic — the pH went *down.* Only one question left . . .

3.   Look at the pCO$_2$. Did it move opposite from the pH? The pH went *down*, so we are really asking if the pCO$_2$ went *up.* Well, did it? No. Since the pH and pCO$_2$ did *not* move in *opposite* directions, the primary underlying problem is *metabolic*.

Putting everything together, the patient has a *metabolic acidosis* with mild concomitant hypoxia. Now lets *prove* that we're right, rather than memorizing. Here, we'll use the mathematical technique of proc by "assuming the opposite" and discovering we were right the first time.

What if we're wrong and the primary problem is *really* respiratory? Well, what would the effect on th pCO₂ be in a primary respiratory situation if the pH were *decreased* by 0.15 units? The pCO₂ should *increase* by 15 mm Hg. Obviously, this is *not* the case, proving that we were correct in the first place. Let's try one more example before discussing compensation . . .

Example 4 — 45-year-old woman who has received NG suction X 36 h and inappropriate fluid-replacement.

Parameter	Patient	Normal
pH	7.56	7.35-7.45
pCO₂	35	35-45 mm Hg (torr)
pO₂	80	> 80 mm Hg (torr)

Now, ask the "three questions":

1.   Look at the pO₂. Is it low?. Seems *OK* to me; be happy and move on to the next question.

2.   Look at the pH. Assuming it's not normal, is it too high or too low? It's *too high*; thus, the patient is alkalotic— the pH went *up*. Only one question left . . .

3.   Look at the pCO₂. Did it move opposite from the pH? The pH went *up,* so we are really asking the pCO₂ went *down.* Well, did it? No way. Since the pH and pCO₂ did *not* move in *opposite* directions, the primary underlying problem is *metabolic*.

Putting everything together, the patient has a *metabolic alkalosis* with no significant hypoxia. Now, le *prove* that we're right, rather than memorizing. Again, let's use the same mathematical technique. Wh if we're wrong and the primary problem is *really* respiratory. Well, what would the effect on the pCO be in a primary respiratory situation if the pH were *increased* by 0.16 units? The pCO₂ should *decreas* by 16 mm Hg. Obviously, this is *not* the case, proving that we were correct originally. Now, let's consider compensation.

Compensation. Rather than present lots of complicated tables to memorize, let's review the rules of compensation, then try a case:

- Respiratory compensation via the lungs for a primary metabolic process is quick (minutes to hours).

- Metabolic compensation via the kidneys for a respiratory process is slower (hours to days).

- Complete compensation is unusual; overcompensation is rare.

Example 5 — 35-year-old female with a known history of diabetes. She complains of nausea and vomiting for two days. The serum pregnancy test is negative. Her respiratory rate is 25/min.

Parameter	Patient	Normal
pH	7.25	**7.35-7.45**
pCO$_2$	20	**35-45 mm Hg (torr)**
pO$_2$	110	**> 80 mm Hg (torr)**

Now, ask the "three questions":

1. Look at the pO$_2$. Is it low?. It's *normal;* not a problem here, so let's move on.

2. Look at the pH. Assuming it's not normal, is it too high or too low? It's *too low*; thus, the patient is acidotic — the pH went *down*. Only one question left . . .

3. Look at the pCO$_2$. Did it move opposite from the pH? The pH went *down*, so we are really asking if the pCO$_2$ went *up*. Well, did it? No. Since the pH and pCO$_2$ did *not* move in *opposite* directions, the primary underlying problem is *metabolic*.

Putting everything together, the patient has a *metabolic acidosis* with no significant hypoxia. Now, lets *prove* that we're right, rather than memorizing. Again, let's use the mathematical technique of proof by "assuming the opposite." What if we're wrong and the primary problem is *really* respiratory? Well, what would the effect on the pCO$_2$ be in a primary respiratory situation if the pH were *decreased* by 0.15 units? The pCO$_2$ should *increase* by 15 mm Hg. Obviously, this is *not* the case, proving that we were correct originally.

But, wait, there's more . . . look at the pCO$_2$. It's low, indicating that in addition to the primary underlying metabolic acidosis, the patient has a *compensatory* respiratory alkalosis. Think about it — if you've got a metabolic acidosis and want to compensate, what would you do? "Blow off" *respiratory* acid. It's really the only acute alternative, since the kidneys won't get rid of the abnormal metabolic acid for a while, right? And, deep sighing ventilations (Kussmaul's respirations) are a common clinical finding in patients with metabolic acidosis from any of a number of causes. These indicate *respiratory*

111

compensation (respiratory alkalosis) for a *metabolic* problem.

If you're up to it, I have a compensation question: Assuming that we could actually identify the exact moment at which the above patient began her respiratory compensation (which is, in reality, nearly impossible), what was her pH *prior* to the onset of respiratory compensation? Give it some thought, then look at the hints below.

If we assume that the pCO_2 was normal (40 mm Hg) prior to the onset of compensation, the question really becomes "what is the effect on the pH of *lowering* the pCO_2 by 20 mm Hg?" The answer, (based on the "happy marriage", is that it should *increase* by 0.2 units. If the pH, with compensation, is now 7.20, we assume it's 0.2 units *higher* than before compensation occurred. Do the math — 7.25 minus 0.20 equals 7.05, the approximate starting pH prior to the onset of respiratory compensation. Since pH is a logarithmic scale (remember, pH = - Log $[H^+]$), a change in pH of 0.2 units translates to a significant decrease in acid content of the patient's blood.

A trip down logarithm row (optional). If the patient in the above example started with a pH of 7.05, she hyperventilated away ("blew off") 20 mm Hg of her pCO_2, raising the pH to 7.25. The question is: by raising the pH from 7.05 to 7.25 (0.2 pH units), how much did the acid level ($[H^+]$) in her blood change? First of all, intuition tells us that the $[H^+]$ must have *decreased*, else the pH wouldn't have increased — agreed? The easiest way to answer the question is using the mathematical formula for pH and to solve for the $[H^+]$:

$$pH = - Log_{10} [H^+]$$

Remember the definition of a logarithm:

$$If\ Log_A\ (B) = X,\ then\ A^X = B$$

So, for each pH (7.05 and 7.25), we can solve for the hydrogen ion concentration, $[H^+]$:

pH = 7.05 (before compensation)	pH = 7.25 (after compensation)
7.05 = - Log_{10} $[H^+]$ *(multiply both sides by -1)*	7.25 = - Log_{10} $[H^+]$ *(multiply both sides by -1)*
$10^{-7.05}$ = $[H^+]$	$10^{-7.25}$ = $[H^+]$
8.9×10^{-8} = $[H^+]$	5.6×10^{-8} = $[H^+]$

Now, compare the $[H^+]$ before and after compensation. After respiratory compensation, the $[H^+]$ level *decreased*, leading to an *increase* in the pH. So, the acid level *decreased* by (8.9 - 5.6)/8.9 = .37 or 37% (remember, the exponents cancel out). **Small *changes in pH reflect relatively* large *changes in $[H^+]$ levels due to the logarithmic scale.***

And, in summary . . . That's all there really is to it. Whether or not a compensatory process is present, you should always use the "three questions" to identify the primary process. Once you've got that issue settled, look for respiratory compensation if the primary process is metabolic. If the primary process is respiratory, look now at the serum electrolytes and the bicarbonate level to determine if a compensatory metabolic process is present.

ASK ONLY THREE QUESTIONS:

1. **Look at the pO_2. Is it low?**

2. **Look at the pH. Which way did it go, up (too high) or down (too low)?**

3. **Look at the pCO_2. Did the pCO_2 move in the *opposite* direction of the pH?**

CHAPTER 8 – CARDIAC ENZYMES AND NATRIURETIC PROTEIN LEVELS

CHAPTER 8 – CARDIAC ENZYMES AND NATRIURETIC PROTEIN LEVELS

CARDIAC ENZYMES

There are several enzymes that are released when heart cells are damaged. A specific, sensitive marker that is present in 1-2 hours after the cardiac muscle injury continues to be sought. Similarly, a marker that effectively *rules out* myocardial ischemia/infarction, especially in the early hours of presentation, has yet to be found.

- **Parameters measured:** CK, CK isozymes, CK-MB isoforms, LDH/LDH isozymes, serum myoglobin, cardiac troponin T/I [**NOTE**: "isozymes" and "isoenzymes" are synonyms]

- **The test in a "nutshell":** Used to help determine the presence or absence of cardiac damage from myocardial infarction; helpful in determining patient risk in acute coronary syndromes

- **Normal values:** Vary widely from lab to lab, depending on the method used

WARNING!!

MUST be used in conjunction with clinical impression, history, and EKG before any definitive conclusions may be reached!! If positive, enzymes may be helpful...if normal, they DO NOT rule out acute MI!! *ALL* results should be reported promptly to the ordering health care provider.

- **Results in a "nutshell":**

NOTE: AST (SGOT) was used in the past as a marker of acute myocardial infarction. It is rarely used any more and mentioned here only for historical interest.

PARAMETER	IMPLICATIONS
CK (CPK)	Nonspecific by itself; requires isozyme determinations.
CK-MB isozyme (CPK-MB isozyme)	Significant elevation relatively specific for acute myocardial damage; normal values, especially early (first 4-6 hours), does **NOT** rule out acute MI.
CK-MB isoforms	Considered experimental; early data look promising to identify early MI; normal values do **NOT** rule out MI.

LDH, LDH isozymes	Somewhat helpful; no longer used by many experts anymore to diagnose myocardial infarction; isozymes essential – LDH, by itself, very nonspecific; normal values do **NOT** rule out MI.
Serum myoglobin	Relatively new; not widely available; highly specific for early diagnosis of myocardial infarction ; normal values do **NOT** rule out MI, though it may be more sensitive than CK-MB.
Cardiac troponin T (troponin I also used)	Some data suggest has higher sensitivity; commercially available rapid assay gives results in 1-20 minutes; normal values do **NOT** rule out MI

- Test details

PARAMETER	IMPLICATIONS
Creatine kinase – **found in heart muscle (CK-MB), skeletal muscle (CK-MM), and brain (CK-BB).**	Creatine kinase is increased in over 90% of myocardial infarctions. However, it can be increased in muscle trauma, physical exertion, postoperatively, convulsions, delirium tremens and other conditions. CK-MB isozyme determinations are necessary in most cases (see below). Time sequence after myocardial infarction • Begins to rise 4-6 hours • Peaks 24 hours • Returns to normal in 3-4 days
CK-MB isozyme – **CK has 3 forms: MB [cardiac], MM [skeletal muscle], and BB [brain]. 15% of CK in cardiac tissue is MB, the rest MM.**	Elevation of CK-MB is relatively specific for acute myocardial damage; normal values, especially early (first 4-6 hours), do **NOT** rule out acute MI. Elevated CK-MB with normal total CK levels = increased risk of acute cardiac events. Peak *not* correlate with infarct size. Serial sampling increases accuracy, but fails to diagnose 10% of AMI patients.

CK subforms – **CK-MM and CK-MB exist in the heart as subforms MM$_3$ and MB$_2$ In the blood, they are converted to MM$_1$ and MB$_1$, respectively. CK-MB isoforms have been used experimentally.**	Only one isoform (CK-MB2) is present in cardiac muscle. CK-MB2 is converted to CK-MB1 in the serum. The normal serum CK-MB2/CK-MB1 ratio (about 1.0) is increased in patients with an AMI. Isoforms may be detectable 1 - 2 hours earlier than CK-MB and may also peak earlier (4 - 6 hours) than CK-MB. The isoform test may reach > 95% sensitivity ~ 6 hours after the onset of chest pain and result in earlier exclusion of an AMI than is presently possible with CK-MB testing (> 95 % sensitivity only after ~ 8 - 10 hours). However, the isoform test requires specialized equipment and is technically difficult to perform. The test is not available at all institutions. Using the CB-MB isoform test as the standard cardiac marker test results in a major increased expense and only decreases the AMI-exclusion threshold from ~ 8 hours (CK-MB) to ~ 6 hours (CK-MB isoforms). Normal values do **NOT** rule out MI.
Serum myoglobin – **oxygen-carrying protein of muscle; released into circulation through capillaries in myocardial injury**	Found in striated muscle. Damage to skeletal or cardiac muscle releases myoglobin into circulation. Highly specific for early diagnosis of myocardial infarction (rises 1-4 hours following symptom onset, peaks 6-9 hr, back to baseline 18-24 hr); serial levels most helpful (doubling within 2 hours = 95% sensitivity and specificity for AMI); normal values do **NOT** rule out MI though low likelihood of AMI if not elevated within 4 h of symptoms. Still fails to detect 5-10% of patients with AMI.

***Cardiac troponin T and I* – muscle regulatory proteins; T (TnT) and I (TnI) are cardiac-specific.**	Many consider the cardiac troponins I and T the preferred markers for the diagnosis of myocardial injury. These are contractile proteins of the myofibril. The cardiac isoforms are very specific for cardiac injury and are not present in serum from healthy people. TnT is elevated in acute coronary syndromes *and* AMI. Take 4-6 hours to rise but remain elevated for a week or more (good *late* marker). Though not diagnostic for AMI, elevated levels correlate with cardiac death or AMI in persons with acute coronary syndromes. TnI is similar, but may be more accurate. Negative values do **NOT** rule out MI and are of little prognostic significance. Bedside tests available. **NOTE**: elevation of TnT or TnI is absolutely indicative of cardiac damage, but this can occur as a result of causes other than MI. Myocarditis, coronary artery spasm from cocaine, severe cardiac failure, cardiac trauma from surgery or motor vehicle accident, and pulmonary embolus can cause cardiac damage with an accompanying elevation of cardiac troponin(s).

Lactic dehydrogenase (LDH) – LDH is found in heart muscle, skeletal muscle, liver, erythrocytes, kidney, and some neoplasms.	LDH is increased in over 90% of myocardial infarctions. However, it can be increased in diseases of any of the organs mentioned in the first column or hemolysis. Time sequence of LD after myocardial infarction: • Begins to rise 24 hours • Peaks in 3 days • Returns to normal in 8-9 days LDH isoenzymes: • LD1 - heart, erythrocytes, renal cortex • LD2 - reticuloendothelial system • LD3 - lung tissue • LD4 - placenta, kidney, pancreas • LD5 - skeletal muscle, liver Reversal of LD1/ LD2 ratio is characteristic of an acute myocardial infarction; with an 80-85% sensitivity.

NATRIURETIC PROTEIN LEVELS

- **Parameters measured:**   Atrial natriuretic protein (ANP), brain natriuretic protein (BNP)

- **The test in a "nutshell":**   Levels of both ANP and BNP are elevated in response to stretching of the ventricles, both left and right. Both are often elevated in heart failure, but other conditions also elevate these proteins, especially the BNP. With limitations, the BNP test is helpful in screening patients for asymptomatic left ventricular dysfunction, and in differentiating causes of dyspnea.

- **Normal values:**

Parameter	Normal value (adults)
Atrial natriuretic protein (ANP)	**36 pg/mL**
Brain natriuretic protein (BNP)	**< 100 pg/mL**

PANIC VALUES!!

BNP > 500 pg/mL

- **Results in a "nutshell":**

PARAMETER	IMPLICATIONS
Atrial natriuretic protein (ANP)	Elevated in response to volume stretch of the heart, most often due to heart failure. Not detectable by current tests early enough to help in screening or early diagnosis. Used to prioritize patients for cardiac transplant.
Brain natriuretic protein (BNP)	Elevated in response to volume stretch of the heart, often due to heart failure, though other diseases can also cause mild to moderate elevations. Elevations > 500 pg/mL are usually due to left ventricular systolic dysfunction (heart failure).

- **Test Details**

1. Four natriuretic proteins have been discovered – atrial natriuretic protein (ANP), brain natriuretic protein (BNP), CNP, and DNP. The last two (CNP, DNP) are not acronyms – they were named in the order discovered.

2. All four natriuretic proteins are released from the heart in response to volume stretch. Though the specifics vary between them, all have the same general functions:

    - Sodium diuresis
    - Vasodilation
    - Reversal of collagen production

    Thus, the effects of the natriuretic proteins are *opposite* to those of the renin-angiotensin-aldosterone system (salt and water retention, vasoconstriction, production of collagen).

3. Fluid retention, as a result of heart failure (HF), leads to volume stretch of the heart and release of the natriuretic proteins – an attempt of the body to compensate for volume overload. In the early stages of HF, this works. However, as HF becomes more progressive, the body's natural defense system (i.e., the natriuretic proteins) are no longer effective. The heart, though, continues to manufacture them as long as volume stretch (HF) continues. Thus, levels of the various natriuretic proteins should be an indicator of the level of cardiac dysfunction.

4.   Though CNP and DNP are known to exist, their exact role in normal fluid homeostasis and in HF are not clear. They will not be discussed here.

5.   ANP levels are fairly insensitive unless the patient has clinically advanced disease. By the time ANP can be detected in a laboratory, the patient will have obvious HF, generally far-advanced. In fact, ANP levels are generally only used clinically to prioritize patients on heart transplant waiting lists.

6.   BNP levels rise early in HF, and in relative proportion to the degree of ventricular dysfunction.[16] Originally, BNP levels were thought to be very sensitive for left ventricular (LV) systolic dysfunction. More recent research, however, has confirmed that other entities can also increase BNP levels. These include: diastolic dysfunction, right ventricular failure, pulmonary embolus, and chronic obstructive pulmonary disease (COPD). Thus, our ability to use BNP levels to determine whether or not a patient has LV systolic dysfunction as a cause of his or her symptoms is limited.

7.   A bedside test for BNP is now available (Triage BNP kit®). The results can be obtained quickly and in a relatively cost-effective manner.

8.   Despite its limitations, recent data support the following clinical uses of BNP levels:

   •   Large elevations (> 500 pg/mL) are usually due to heart failure, especially if the clinical picture fits.

   •   Asymptomatic patients who are at high risk for HF (i.e., diabetics, persons with hypertension) with BNP levels of < 50 pg/dL are *extremely unlikely* to have significant LV dysfunction on either echocardiogram or angiogram. Most experts feel that, in this group, testing beyond BNP levels is not necessary.

   •   Dyspneic patients with BNP levels of < 50 pg/dL are *very unlikely* to have significant LV dysfunction as the cause of their dyspnea. On the other hand, mild elevations (100 - 300 pg/mL) may be due to HF, COPD, or pulmonary embolism – so, unless the BNP level is significantly elevated, high levels are less helpful in discerning the cause of dyspnea than are low levels.

   •   There are no significant studies to date that provide guidelines for patients with BNP levels between 50-100 pg/ml.

9.   Though not widely available, amino terminal-pro-BNP (NT-proBNP) levels are thought by some to be more sensitive than BNP alone.[17]

CHAPTER 9 – PREGNANCY TESTS

CHAPTER 9 – PREGNANCY TESTS

Urine pregnancy tests, unless specific for the ß-subunit of human chorionic gonadotropin (ß-hCG), are notoriously unreliable. False positive tests are common, so results must be confirmed with a serum test. Most clinicians skip the urine test (with the aforementioned exception) and simply perform a serum pregnancy test.

- **Parameters measured:**   Serum or urine ß-subunit of human chorionic gonadotropin (ß-hCG)

- **The test in a "nutshell":**   Measures presence or absence of ß-hCG (**qualitative**) in serum or urine; the **quantitative test** measures the actual level, usually in the serum.

- **Normal values:**

  ‣ **Qualitative** – negative (not pregnant)

  ‣ **Quantitative** – males < 2.5 IU/L; nonpregnant females < 5.0 IU/L, postmenopausal females < 9.0 IU/L; pregnancy:

Weeks Past LMP	ß-hCG IU/L
3	0-5
4	3-426
5	18-7,340
6	1,080-56,600
7-8	7,650-229,000
9-12	25,700-288,000
13-16	13,300-253,000
17-24	4,060-65,400
25-40	3,640-117,000

- **Results in a "nutshell":**   indicates pregnancy (positive within 3 days of implantation, molar pregnancy, or ectopic pregnancy; may remain elevated for weeks after delivery; even longer after D&C for termination of pregnancy or hysterectomy for molar removal. Also elevated in testicular tumors.

- ■ **Basic physiology**

  - ▸ ß-hCG produced by **trophoblast** (outer layer of developing embryonic mass); transported via blood to the ovaries, causing the **corpus luteum** to remain functional.

  - ▸ Corpus luteum (in ovary) secretes **estrogen** and **progesterone** to maintain the pregnanc

  - ▸ The **placenta** forms from the trophoblast and uterine tissue; it begins to secrete estroger and progesterone.

  - ▸ The placenta produces sufficient estrogen and progesterone by the 3rd month to maintai pregnancy; the corpus luteum is no longer needed and degenerates.

  - ▸ Thus, ß-hCG levels increase early following implantation, reaching a maximum concentration near the end of the first trimester; they then decrease to a low level thereafter.

- ■ **Test details**

Specificity, sensitivity, and persistence of elevation

  - ▸ The qualitative ß-hCG test is sensitive down to 1-3 IU/L; it is the **most specific and most sensitive test** for the detection of early pregnancy, ectopic pregnancy, or threatene abortion. Levels can usually be detected within 3-10 days of implantation.

  - ▸ ß-hCG levels may be detected up to 3-4 weeks following normal delivery or terminatio of pregnancy..

  - ▸ ß-hCG may take anywhere from 11 to 200+ days to disappear following evacuation of a molar pregnancy.

  - ▸ Various germ cell neoplasms also produce ß-hCG (choriocarcinoma, hydatidiform mole germinal testicular tumors).

Interpretation of results – quantitative levels

  - ▸ **Increased** in pregnancy, hydatidiform mole, choriocarcinoma, seminoma, ovarian and testicular teratomas, multiple pregnancy, other neoplasms (stomach, pancreas, lung, colon, liver), malignant melanoma. Absence of a gestational sac on routine abdominal ultrasound with serum ß-hCG > 6500 IU/L suggests ectopic.

▸ **Decreased** (lower than expected for age of pregnancy) are found in threatened abortion and ectopic pregnancy. Quantitative levels should double every 2-3 days in normal intrauterine pregnancy.

Potential confounders...

▸ <u>Patients cannot reliably predict</u> on their own whether or not they are pregnant – there is at least a 10% chance of the patient being incorrect when she states she is not pregnant.[18]

▸ Rarely, a patient can have a <u>heterotopic pregnancy</u> – concomitant intrauterine and ectopic pregnancy.[19]

▸ Of patients who have undergone <u>tubal ligation</u> for sterilization, 0.5% will still become pregnant. Of these, 50% will develop an ectopic. There have been several reported cases of <u>ectopic pregnancy developing in women who have undergone hysterectomy</u>. It is felt that a fistula develops between the vagina and abdominal cavity, allowing for fertilization to occur if ovulation is present.

CHAPTER 10 – CLOTTING FUNCTION TESTS
PARAMETERS MEASURED
THE TEST IN A "NUTSHELL"
NORMAL VALUES
THERAPEUTIC VALUES
PANIC VALUES
RESULTS IN A "NUTSHELL"
BASIC PHYSIOLOGY – THE COAGULATION CASCADE
TEST DETAILS

CHAPTER 10 – CLOTTING FUNCTION TESTS

■ **Parameters measured:** Protime (PT), international normalized ratio (INR), partial thromboplastin time (PTT); also see platelet count and bleeding time (under CBC, earlier). The APTT (activated PTT) is a more sensitive version of the PTT used primarily to monitor heparin anticoagulant therapy.

■ **The test in a "nutshell":** Used to determine the adequacy of the body's blood coagulation system (intrinsic and extrinsic clotting systems); may be abnormal in liver disease, DIC, cancer, or specific blood conditions (such as hemophilia). Commonly ordered to monitor anticoagulation therapy, to evaluate bleeding, to evaluate liver function.

■ **Normal values:**

Protime (PT)	11.0-13.0 seconds
P/C ratio	1.3 - 1.5
International normalized ratio (INR)	1.0 - 1.5
Partial thromboplastin time (PTT)	30-45 seconds

■ **Therapeutic values:**

▸ **PT** – during warfarin (Coumadin®) therapy there are two systems now used; the older system compares the ratio of the patients PT to the laboratory control:

P/C ratio = Patient's PT/Control PT

Using this system, adequate anticoagulation is a PC ratio between 1.3 - 1.5. A newer system, the **International Normalized Ratio (INR)** is a comparison of the patient's PT to an international standard:

INR = Patients PT/International Reference Thromboplastin

INR is felt to be a more sensitive way to monitor oral anticoagulation. It is reproducible between various laboratories, unlike the PT, which is lab specific (depends on the method used to perform the test). The accepted range for INR varies, depending on the degree of oral anticoagulation desired:

Condition (normal = 1.0 - 1.5)	Preferred INR Range
Preoperative hip surgery	2.0-3.0
Prevention of systemic embolism in pts with atrial fibrillation	2.0-3.0
Recurrent systemic embolism	3.0-4.5
Prevention of recurrent deep vein thrombosis (2 or more episodes)	2.5-4.0
Cardiac stents	3.0-4.5
Prevention of arterial thrombosis including mechanical heart valves	3.0-4.5

▶ **PTT** – during heparin therapy (full intravenous dosing), usually maintained at 1.5-2.0 times the laboratory control (normal) value.

PANIC FINDINGS!!

P/C ratio > 2.5
PT > 30 seconds
INR > 4.5
APTT or PTT > 100 seconds

■ **Results in a "nutshell":**

PARAMETER	IMPLICATIONS
Protime (PT), International normalized ratio (INR), P/C ratio	Monitors stage II of the clotting process; evaluates clotting ability of prothrombin, fibronogen, factor V, factor VII, and factor X; used to monitor oral anticoagulant (warfarin, Coumadin) therapy. Goal is to keep P/C ratio 1.3-1.5 or INR within range for the specific condition (see table above).
Partial thromboplastin time (PTT)	Detects abnormalities of both Stage I and Stage II; APTT is a more sensitive version of PTT, often used to monitor heparin therapy. Maintain at 1.5-2.0 times the control value.

■ **Basic physiology – The Coagulation Cascade**

Clotting proceeds in three stages:

▶ **Stage 1** – formation of **prothrombinase**; two pathways involved, but may be inter-related:

• **Extrinsic clotting pathway** – begins with chemicals outside or extrinsic to the blood; damaged tissues release a mixture of lipoproteins and phospholipids called **tissue factors (TF**; also known as **thromboplastin** or **factor III**). In the presence of calcium, TF activates **factor VII** to **factor VIIa**. Factor VIIa activates **factor X** (to **factor Xa**). Factor Xa and **factor V** combine on the platelet surface with calcium ions and platelet phospholipids to form **prothrombinase**.

• **Intrinsic clotting pathway** – begins with chemicals that are inside or intrinsic to the blood; damage to blood vessels exposes collagen; as plasma **factor XII** comes into contact with collagen, it is activated; activated factor XII (**XIIa**) activates **factor XI** forming **factor XIa** which activates **factor IX**. **Activated factor IX (IXa)** joins with **factor VIII**, platelet phospholipids, and calcium ions to activate **factor X (factor Xa)**. Factor Xa and **factor V** combine on the platelet surface with calcium ions and platelet phospholipids to form **prothrombinase**.

So, in Stage I, the end result is that factor X is activated (by the intrinsic system, the extrinsic system, or both). Activated factor X (Xa) combines with factor V, calcium, and platelet phospholipids on the platelet surface to form prothrombinase...

▶ **Stage 2** --conversion of **prothrombin** to **thrombin** by prothrombinase.

▶ **Stage 3** – Conversion of soluble **fibrinogen** to insoluble **fibrin**. Accomplished by prothrombinase. The final fibrin clot is stabilized by activated **factor XIII (XIIIa)**.

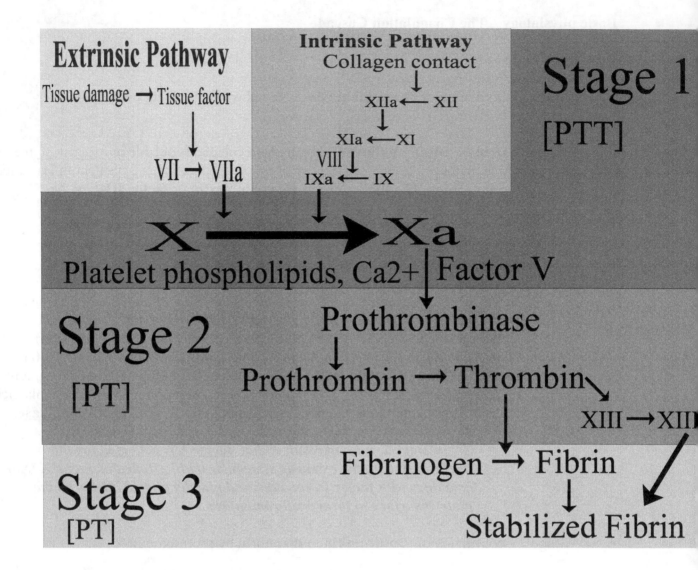

■ **Test details**

Protime (PT)/International normalized ratio (INR

▸ Oral anticoagulants work indirectly by interfering with the liver's formation of the **vitamin-K dependent clotting factors** (II, VII, IX, X). They competitively inhibit the effects of vitamin K on gamma carboxylation of the proteins; since the inhibition is competitive, it may be overcome with vitamin K supplementation or factor replacement (usually with fresh frozen plasma).

▸ **Increased** with deficiency of vitamin-K dependent clotting factors (II, VII, IX, X), vitamin K deficiency, liver disease, anticoagulant therapy, biliary obstruction, salicylate intoxication, DIC, lupus (circulating anticoagulant interferes with extrinsic pathway).

- **Decreased** by ovarian hyperfunction, regional enteritis.

- **Not affected** by polycythemia vera, Hemophilia A (factor VIII), von Willebrand's disease, platelet disorders.

Partial thromboplastin time (PTT)

- Screens primarily for defects in the **intrinsic clotting system**, but will also detect some of the extrinsic system.

- **Prolonged** in all congenital deficiencies of intrinsic system coagulation factors (e.g., Hemophilia A and hemophilia B), heparin therapy, warfarin therapy (sometimes), vitamin K deficiency (sometimes), liver disease, DIC.

- **Shortened** in extensive cancer (where liver **NOT** involved), immediately after acute hemorrhage.

- **Heparin** is a direct anticoagulant that binds to **antithrombin III (AT III)**; together the complex inhibits the generation of thrombin.

CHAPTER 11 – LIPID TESTS AND C-REACTIVE PROTEIN (CRP)

LIPID TESTS
> PARAMETERS MEASURED
> THE TEST IN A "NUTSHELL"
> NORMAL VALUES
> PANIC VALUES
> RESULTS IN A "NUTSHELL"
> TEST DETAILS

C-REACTIVE PROTEIN (CRP)
> PARAMETERS MEASURED
> THE TEST IN A "NUTSHELL"
> NORMAL VALUES
> PANIC VALUES
> RESULTS IN A "NUTSHELL"
> TEST DETAILS

CHAPTER 11 – LIPID TESTS AND C-REACTIVE PROTEIN (CRP)

LIPID TESTS

■ **Parameters measured:** Cholesterol, LDL-C (low-density, "bad cholesterol"), HDL-C (high-density, "good cholesterol"), triglycerides.

■ **The test in a "nutshell":** Helpful in screening for increased risk of coronary artery disease (atherosclerosis), peripheral vascular disease, and stroke

■ **Normal values:**

Parameter	Normal value (adults)
Cholesterol	< 200 mg/dL
LDL-C	< 100 mg/dL
HDL-C	40 - 60 mg/dL
Triglycerides	< 150 mg/dL

PANIC VALUES!!

Cholesterol > 240 mg/dL
LDL-C > 160 mg/dL
HDL-C <40 mg/dL
Triglycerides > 500 mg/dL

- **Results in a "nutshell":**

PARAMETER	IMPLICATIONS
Cholesterol	Elevations of total cholesterol associated with increased risk of cardiovascular disease. Subtype (LDL-C, HDL-C) levels are more important than the total cholesterol level alone.
LDL-C	Elevations are a major cause of cardiovascular disease; reducing levels significantly decrease risks.
HDL-C	Decreased levels are associated with an increased risk of cardiovascular disease. Increasing levels significantly decreases risks. It is thought that this form of cholesterol somehow helps the body eliminate the LDL-C ("bad") cholesterol.
Triglycerides	Elevated levels are an independent risk factor for cardiovascular disease.

- **Test details – LIPID DISORDERS** *(enrichment)*

[A]   Definition

Dyslipidemia refers to any abnormality of the blood lipids (fats). Hyperlipidemia is an elevation of lipids in the bloodstream. These lipids are transported in the blood as part of large molecules called lipoproteins – molecules of fat and cholesterol linked to protein.

[B]   Types of Lipoproteins

These are the five major families of blood (plasma) lipoproteins:

- Chylomicrons – composed of triglycerides, cholesterol, and protein. Chylomicrons, the largest lipoproteins, carry exogenous triglyceride from the intestine via the thoracic duct to the venous system. In the capillaries of adipose and muscle tissue, 90% of chylomicron triglyceride is removed by a specific group of lipases (fat-breakdown enzymes). The remnants of chylomicrons, depleted of most of their triglycerides but still containing cholesterol and protein, travel in the blood to the liver. Here, they are used as fuel or precursors to form other molecules. If these remnants are not immediately needed by the liver, they are packaged into VLDLs (see below) and transported in the blood to the adipose and muscle tissue. Here, the triglycerides are removed and stored in lipid droplets within adipocytes or metabolized for energy in the myocytes.

- Very low-density lipoproteins (VLDL) – composed of cholesterol and triglycerides, with little protein. VLDL carries triglyceride from the liver to fat cells where it is stored or muscle cells where it is used for energy (see above).

- Intermediate-density lipoproteins (IDL) – the same lipases that act on chylomicrons quickly degrade endogenous triglyceride in VLDL, giving rise to intermediate density lipoproteins (IDL) that are shorn of much of their triglyceride and surface proteins. Most of the IDLs are metabolized to LDL or are taken up by the liver.

- Low-density lipoproteins (LDL) – rich in cholesterol, LDLs carry cholesterol to extrahepatic tissues that have specific receptors (apoB-100). These receptors mediate the uptake of cholesterol into cells. This is also the form of cholesterol that is taken up by blood vessels, leading to atherosclerosis (hardening of the arteries). Thus, LDL-cholesterol is termed "bad cholesterol."

- High-density lipoproteins (HDL) – HDLs begin in the liver and small intestine as small, protein-rich particles that contain relatively little cholesterol. However, HDLs are rich in enzymes that convert tissue cholesterol into a form that can be transported by them to the liver. Here the cholesterol is unloaded and metabolized to bile salts. HDLs, thus, participate in what has been termed reverse cholesterol transport – moving cholesterol from the organs (including arteries) to the liver, where it is metabolized. This has a beneficial (anti-atherosclerotic) effect. Thus, HDL-cholesterol is termed "good cholesterol."

[C]   Classification of Hyperlipidemia

When hyperlipidemia is defined in terms of a class or classes of elevated lipoproteins in the blood, the term hyperlipoproteinemia is used. There are several genetically-determined syndromes that involve abnormalities of various classes of lipoproteins. All of these syndromes, to one degree or another, place the affected individual at an increased risk for cardiovascular disease, especially stroke and myocardial infarction (MI; heart attack). In common medical practice, many patients arc not diagnosed and treated based on these classifications. Most clinicians and researchers look at two general terms:

- Hypercholesterolemia is the term for high cholesterol levels in the blood.

- Hypertriglyceridemia refers to high triglyceride levels in the blood.

When evaluating patients in terms of their cardiovascular risks, clinicians measure four parameters:

- The total blood cholesterol level
- The total blood triglycerides level
- The amount of HDL-cholesterol
- The amount of LDL-cholesterol

135

[D]   ATP III Guidelines

The Third Report of the National Cholesterol Education Program (NCEP) Expert Panel on Detection, Evaluation, and Treatment of High Blood Cholesterol in Adults (Adult Treatment Panel III, or ATP III) presents the NCEP's updated clinical guidelines for cholesterol testing and management. The ATP III guidelines provide detailed information on topic areas such as classification of lipids and lipoproteins, coronary heart disease (CHD) risk assessment, lifestyle interventions, drug treatment, specific dyslipidemias, and adherence issues. Recommendations for special populations such as patients with CHD, patients at high risk for developing CHD, patients with diabetes, women, older Americans, young adults, and racial and ethnic groups are provided.[20]

The information here is based on the Executive Summary of the above-referenced document, which contains treatment recommendations derived from the evidence-based full ATP III report.[21]

[1]   New Features

The ATP III report is the third in a series published for clinical management of high blood lipids. New features in the current report include:

1.   Focus on multiple risk factors

- Raises persons with diabetes without CHD, most of whom display multiple risk factors, to the risk level of CHD risk equivalent.
- Uses Framingham projections of 10-year absolute CHD risk (i.e., the percent probability of having a CHD event in 10 years) to identify certain patients with multiple (2+) risk factors for more intensive treatment.
- Identifies persons with multiple metabolic risk factors (metabolic syndrome) as candidates for intensified therapeutic lifestyle changes.

2.   Modifications of lipid and lipoprotein classification

- Identifies LDL cholesterol <100 mg/dL as optimal.
- Raises categorical low HDL cholesterol from <35 mg/dL to <40 mg/dL because the latter is a better measure of a depressed HDL.
- Lowers the triglyceride classification cutpoints to give more attention to moderate elevations.

3.   Support for implementation

- Recommends a complete lipoprotein profile (total cholesterol, LDL cholesterol, HDL cholesterol, and triglycerides) as the preferred initial test, rather than screening for total cholesterol and HDL alone.
- Encourages use of plant stanols/sterols and viscous (soluble) fiber as therapeutic dietary options to enhance lowering of LDL cholesterol.
- Presents strategies for promoting adherence to therapeutic lifestyle changes and drug therapies.

136

- Recommends treatment beyond LDL lowering for persons with triglycerides ≥ 200 mg/dL.

[2] Desired Goals, in General

Elevated LDL cholesterol is a major cause of coronary heart disease (CHD). In addition, recent clinical trials robustly show that LDL-lowering therapy reduces risk for CHD. As a result, the primary goals of therapy and the cutpoints for initiating treatment are stated in terms of LDL.

In all adults aged 20 years or older, a fasting lipoprotein profile (total cholesterol, LDL cholesterol, high density lipoprotein [HDL] cholesterol, and triglyceride) should be obtained once every 5 years. If the testing opportunity is nonfasting, only the values for total cholesterol and HDL cholesterol will be usable. In such a case, if total cholesterol is ≥ 200 mg/dL or HDL is <40 mg/dL, a followup lipoprotein profile is needed for appropriate management based on LDL.

The **TABLE** below summarizes the desired laboratory results:

LDL Cholesterol
<100 Optimal
100-129 Near optimal/above optimal
130-159 Borderline high
160-189 High
≥190 Very high
Total Cholesterol
<200 Desirable
200-239 Borderline high
≥240 High
HDL Cholesterol
<40 Low
≥60 High

[3] Modification of LDL Cholesterol (LDL-C) Goals

[a] Major Risk Factors

The above LDL-C goals are modified, depending upon a given patient's individual risk for CHD. Major risk factors, as used in ATP III, include:

- Cigarette smoking
- Hypertension (BP ≥ 140/90 mm Hg or on antihypertensive medication)

- Low HDL cholesterol (<40 mg/dL) [HDL cholesterol ≥60 mg/dL counts as a "negative" risk factor; its presence removes one risk factor from the total count]
- Family history of premature CHD (CHD in male first degree relative <55 years; CHD in female first degree relative <65 years)
- Age (men ≥ 45 years; women ≥ 55 years)

Note that diabetes is considered as a separate CHD "risk equivalent" (see below).

[b]   Modified Recommendations

Based on the above risk factors and the number of risk equivalents, the goal LDL cholesterol is modified from the initial recommendations above as follows:

Risk Category	LDL Goal (mg/dl)
CHD and CHD risk equivalents	<100
Multiple (2+) risk factors	<130
Zero to one risk factor	<160

[c]   CHD Risk Equivalents

The category of highest risk consists of known CHD and CHD risk equivalents. The latter carry a risk for major coronary events equal to that of established CHD, i.e., >20% per 10 years (i.e., more than 20 of 100 such individuals will develop CHD or have a recurrent CHD event within 10 years). CHD risk equivalents comprise:

- Other clinical forms of atherosclerotic disease (peripheral arterial disease, abdominal aortic aneurysm, and symptomatic carotid artery disease)
- Diabetes
- Multiple risk factors that confer a 10-year risk for CHD >20%

Diabetes counts as a CHD risk equivalent because it confers a high risk of new CHD within 10 years, in part because of its frequent association with multiple risk factors. Furthermore, because persons with diabetes who experience a myocardial infarction have an unusually high death rate either immediately or in the long term, a more intensive prevention strategy is warranted. Persons with CHD or CHD risk equivalents have the lowest LDL cholesterol goal (<100 mg/dL).

The second category consists of persons with multiple (2+) risk factors in whom 10-year risk for CHD is ≤ 20%. Risk is estimated from Framingham risk scores (see below). The risk factors included in the Framingham calculation of 10-year risk are: age, total cholesterol, HDL cholesterol, systolic blood pressure, treatment for hypertension, and cigarette smoking. The major risk factors listed above, exclusive of elevated LDL cholesterol and *in conjunction with* the Framingham risk score, are used to define the presence of multiple risk factors that modify the

138

goals and cutpoints for LDL-lowering treatment. The LDL cholesterol goal for persons with multiple (2+) risk factors *and* a 10-year risk for CHD ≤ 20% (based on the Framingham calculation) is <130 mg/dL.

The third category consists of persons having 0-1 risk factor; with few exceptions, persons in this category have a 10-year risk <10%. Their LDL cholesterol goal is <160 mg/dL.

> [NOTE: The 2004 Update (summarized below) has lowered the LDL-C goal levels in some patients.]

[4]   The Framingham CHD Risk Score

Framingham scoring divides persons with multiple risk factors into those with 10-year risk for CHD of >20%, 10-20%, and <10%. When 0-1 risk factor is present, Framingham scoring is not necessary because 10-year risk rarely reaches levels for intensive intervention; a very high LDL level in such a person may nevertheless warrant consideration of drug therapy to reduce long-term risk. Total cholesterol is used for 10-year risk assessment because of a larger and more robust Framingham database for total than for LDL cholesterol, but LDL cholesterol is the primary target of therapy.

The **TABLES** below provide the point scores for each component. Total the points, then read the 10-year risk (%) of having CHD from the final **TABLE**.

[a]   Framingham Tables for Men

Age	Points
20-34	-9
35-39	-4
40-44	0
45-49	3
50-54	6
55-59	8
60-64	10
65-69	11
70-74	12
75-79	13

Total cholesterol	Age 20-39	Age 40-49	Age 50-59	Age 60-69	Age 70-79
<160	0	0	0	0	0
160-199	4	3	2	1	0
200-239	7	5	3	1	0
240-279	9	6	4	2	1
≥180	11	8	5	3	1

	Age 20-39	Age 40-49	Age 50-59	Age 60-69	Age 70-79
Nonsmoker	0	0	0	0	0
Smoker	8	5	3	1	1

HDL (mg/dL)	Points
≥60	-1
50-59	0
40-49	1
<40	2

Systolic BP (mm Hg)	If Untreated	If Treated
<120	0	0
120-129	0	1
130-139	1	2
140-159	1	2
≥160	2	3

Point Total	10-Year Risk %
<0	1
0	1
1	1
2	1
3	1
4	1
5	2
6	2
7	3
8	4
9	5
10	6
11	8
12	10
13	12
14	16
15	20
16	25
≥17	≥30

[b]   Framingham Tables for Women

Age	Points
20-34	-7
35-39	-3
40-44	0
45-49	3
50-54	6
55-59	8
60-64	10
65-69	12
70-74	14
75-79	16

Total cholesterol	Age 20-39	Age 40-49	Age 50-59	Age 60-69	Age 70-79
<160	0	0	0	0	0
160-199	4	3	2	1	1
200-239	8	6	4	2	1
240-279	11	8	5	3	2
≥180	13	10	7	4	2

	Age 20-39	Age 40-49	Age 50-59	Age 60-69	Age 70-79
Nonsmoker	0	0	0	0	0
Smoker	9	7	4	2	1

HDL (mg/dL)	Points
≥60	-1
50-59	0
40-49	1
<40	2

Systolic BP (mm Hg)	If Untreated	If Treated
<120	0	0
120-129	1	3
130-139	2	4
140-159	3	5
≥160	4	6

Point Total	10-Year Risk %
<9	<1
9	1
10	1
11	1
12	1
13	2
14	2
15	3
16	4
17	5
18	6
19	8
20	11
21	14
22	17
23	22
24	27
≥ 25	≥ 30

[5]   The Metabolic Syndrome

Many persons have a constellation of major risk factors, life-habit risk factors, and emerging risk factors that constitute a condition called the *metabolic syndrome*. Factors characteristic of the metabolic syndrome are abdominal obesity, atherogenic dyslipidemia (elevated triglyceride, small LDL particles, low HDL cholesterol), raised blood pressure, insulin resistance (with or without glucose intolerance), and prothrombotic and proinflammatory states. ATP III recognizes the metabolic syndrome as a secondary target of risk-reduction therapy, after the primary target—LDL cholesterol.

The metabolic syndrome represents a constellation of lipid and nonlipid risk factors of metabolic origin. This syndrome is closely linked to a generalized metabolic disorder called *insulin resistance* in which the normal actions of insulin are impaired. Excess body fat (particularly abdominal obesity) and physical inactivity promote the development of insulin resistance, but some individuals also are genetically predisposed to insulin resistance.

The risk factors of the metabolic syndrome are highly concordant; in aggregate they enhance risk for CHD at any given LDL cholesterol level. For purposes of ATP III, the diagnosis of the metabolic syndrome is made when three or more of the risk determinants shown in the **TABLE** below are present. These determinants include a combination of categorical and borderline risk factors that can be readily measured in clinical practice.

Risk Factor	Defining Level
Abdominal Obesity	Waist Circumference
Men	>102 cm (>40 in)
Women	>88 cm (35 in)
Triglycerides	≥150 mg/dL
HDL Cholesterol	
Men	<40 mg/dL
Women	<50 mg/dL
Blood Pressure	≥130/≥85 mm Hg
Fasting Glucose	≥110 mg/dL

Management of the metabolic syndrome has a two-fold objective: (1) to reduce underlying causes (i.e., obesity and physical inactivity), and (2) to treat associated nonlipid and lipid risk factors.

[a] Management of Underlying Causes of the Metabolic Syndrome

First-line therapies for all lipid and nonlipid risk factors associated with the metabolic syndrome are weight reduction and increased physical activity, which will effectively reduce all of these risk factors. Therefore, after appropriate control of LDL cholesterol, TLC should stress weight reduction and physical activity if the metabolic syndrome is present.

Weight control. In ATP III overweight and obesity are recognized as major, underlying risk factors for CHD and identified as direct targets of intervention. Weight reduction will enhance LDL lowering and reduce all of the risk factors of the metabolic syndrome.

Physical activity. Physical inactivity is likewise a major, underlying risk factor for CHD. It augments the lipid and nonlipid risk factors of the metabolic syndrome. It further may enhance risk by impairing cardiovascular fitness and coronary blood flow. Regular physical activity reduces very low density lipoprotein (VLDL) levels, raises HDL cholesterol, and in some persons, lowers LDL levels. It also can lower blood pressure, reduce insulin resistance, and favorably influence cardiovascular function. Thus, ATP III recommends that regular physical activity become a routine component in management of high serum cholesterol.

[b] Specific Treatment of Lipid and Non-Lipid Risk Factors

Beyond the underlying risk factors, therapies directed against the lipid and nonlipid risk factors of the metabolic syndrome will reduce CHD risk. These include treatment of hypertension, use of aspirin in patients with CHD to reduce the prothrombotic state (guidelines for aspirin use in primary prevention have not been firmly established), and treatment of elevated triglycerides and low HDL cholesterol as discussed below.

[6] LDL-Lowering Therapy in Three Risk Categories

The two major modalities of LDL-lowering therapy are *therapeutic lifestyle changes* (TLC) and *drug therapy*. The **TABLE** below defines LDL cholesterol goals and cutpoints for initiation of TLC and for drug consideration for persons with three categories of risk: CHD and CHD risk equivalents; multiple (2+) risk factors (10-year risk 10-20% and <10%); and 0-1 risk factor.

Risk Category	LDL Goal	LDL Level at Which to Institute TLC	LDL Level at Which to Consider Drug Therapy
CHD or CHD Risk Equivalents (10-yr risk > 20%)	<100 mg/dL	≥100 mg/dL	≥130 mg/dL (100-129 mg/dL, drug optional)
2+ Risk Factors (10-year risk ≤20%)	<130 mg/dL	≥130 mg/dL	10-year risk 10-20%: ≥130 mg/dL 10-year risk <10%: ≥160 mg/dL
0-1 Risk Factor	<160 mg/dL	≥160 mg/dL	≥190 mg/dL (160-189 mg/dL, drug optional)

[7] Therapeutic Lifestyle Changes (TLC)

ATP III recommends a multifaceted lifestyle approach to reduce risk for CHD. This approach is designated *therapeutic lifestyle changes (TLC)*. Its essential features are:

- Reduced intakes of saturated fats (<7% of total calories) and cholesterol (<200 mg per day)
- Therapeutic options for enhancing LDL lowering such as plant stanols/sterols (2 g/day) and increased viscous (soluble) fiber (10-25 g/day)
- Weight reduction
- Increased physical activity

[8] Drug Therapy

[a] Primary Prevention

A portion of the population whose short-term or long-term risk for CHD is high will require LDL-lowering drugs in addition to TLC to reach the designated goal for LDL cholesterol. When drugs are prescribed, attention to TLC should always be maintained and reinforced. Currently available drugs that affect lipoprotein metabolism and their major characteristics are listed in the

TABLE below. Note that active or chronic liver disease is a relative or absolute contraindication for most of these agents.

Drugs	Effect	Side Effects	Clinical Trial Results
HMG CoA reductase inhibitors (statins)*	LDL ↓ HDL ↑ TG ↓	Myopathy; increased liver enzymes	Reduced major coronary events, CHD deaths, need for coronary procedures, stroke, and total mortality
Bile acid sequestrants†	LDL ↓ HDL ↑ TG – or ↑	Gastrointestinal distress, constipation, decreased absorption of some other drugs	Reduced major coronary events and CHD deaths
Nicotinic acid‡	LDL ↓ HDL ↑ TG ↓	Flushing, hyperglycemia, gout, upper GI distress, liver toxicity	Reduced major coronary events and possibly, total mortality
Fibric acids¤	LDL ↓ HDL ↑ TG ↓	Dyspepsia, gallstones, myopathy, unexplained sudden death (in one study)	Reduced major coronary events
Cholesterol absorption blockers¤¤	LDL ↓ HDL ↑ TG ↓	Diarrhea, abdominal pain, sinusitis	Additive benefits when combined with a statin

* = Lovastatin (Mevacor®, 20-80 mg), pravastatin (Pravachol®, 20-40 mg), simvastatin (Zocor®, 20-80 mg), fluvastatin (Lescol®, 20-80 mg), atorvastatin (Lipitor®, 10-80 mg); statins inhibit an enzyme, HMG- CoA reductase, that controls the rate of cholesterol production in the body. These drugs lower cholesterol by slowing down the production of cholesterol and by increasing the liver's ability to remove the LDL-cholesterol already in the blood.

† = Cholestyramine (Questran®, 4-16 g), colestipol (Colestid®, 5-20 g), colesevelam (Welchol®, 2.6-3.8 g); bile acid sequestrants bind with cholesterol-containing bile acids in the intestines and are then eliminated in the stool. The usual effect of bile acid sequestrants is to lower LDL-cholesterol by about 10 to 20 percent.

‡ = Immediate release (crystalline) nicotinic acid (1.5-3 g), extended release nicotinic acid (Niaspan®) (1-2 g), sustained release nicotinic acid (1-2 g). Nicotinic acid or niacin, the water-soluble B vitamin, improves all lipoproteins when given in doses well above the vitamin requirement. Nicotinic acid lowers total cholesterol, LDL-cholesterol, and triglyceride levels, while raising HDL-cholesterol levels. Nicotinamide, another form of

146

the vitamin niacin, does not lower cholesterol levels and should not be used in the place of nicotinic acid.

¤ = Gemfibrozil (Lopid®, 600 mg BID), fenofibrate (Tricor®, 200 mg), clofibrate (Atromid-S®, 1000 mg BID). The cholesterol-lowering drugs called fibrates are primarily effective in lowering triglycerides and, to a lesser extent, in increasing HDL-cholesterol levels. Gemfibrozil, the fibrate most widely used in the United States, can be very effective for patients with high triglyceride levels. However, it is not very effective for lowering LDL- cholesterol.

¤¤ = Ezetimibe (Zetia®; 10 mg once daily); the newest of the "cholesterol" drugs, ezetimibe somehow interferes with the absorption of cholesterol in the intestine. As a result, LDL-C and TG levels fall, while HDL-C levels tend to rise modestly. These drugs are effective as monotherapy but when combined with statins, lead to very impressive synergistic effects.[22]

[b]   Secondary Prevention

For persons with CHD and CHD risk equivalents, the goal is to attain an LDL cholesterol level <100 mg/dL. Most CHD patients will need LDL lowering drug therapy. Other lipid risk factors may also warrant consideration of drug treatment. Whether or not lipid-modifying drugs are used, nonlipid risk factors require attention and favorable modification.

In persons admitted to the hospital for a major coronary event, LDL cholesterol should be measured on admission or within 24 hours. This value can be used for treatment decisions. In general, persons hospitalized for a coronary event or procedure should be discharged on drug therapy if the LDL cholesterol is ≥130 mg/dL. If the LDL is 100–129 mg/dL, clinical judgment should be used in deciding whether to initiate drug treatment at discharge, recognizing that LDL cholesterol levels begin to decline in the first few hours after an event and are significantly decreased by 24-48 hours and may remain low for many weeks. Thus, the initial LDL cholesterol level obtained in the hospital may be substantially lower than is usual for the patient.

Some authorities hold drug therapy should be initiated whenever a patient hospitalized for a CHD-related illness is found to have an LDL cholesterol >100 mg/dL. Initiation of drug therapy at the time of hospital discharge has two advantages. First, at that time patients are particularly motivated to undertake and adhere to risk-lowering interventions; and second, failure to initiate indicated therapy early is one of the causes of a large "treatment gap," because outpatient followup is often less consistent and more fragmented.

[9] **Management of Specific Dyslipidemias**

[a] **Very High LDL Cholesterol (≥190 mg/dL)**

Persons with very high LDL cholesterol usually have genetic forms of hypercholesterolemia: monogenic familial hypercholesterolemia, familial defective apolipoprotein B, and polygenic hypercholesterolemia. Early detection of these disorders through cholesterol testing in young adults is needed to prevent premature CHD. Family testing is important to identify similarly affected relatives. These disorders often require combined drug therapy (statin + bile acid sequestrant) to achieve the goals of LDL-lowering therapy.

[b] **Elevated Serum Triglycerides**

[i] **Causes**

Recent meta-analyses of prospective studies indicate that elevated triglycerides are also an independent risk factor for CHD. Factors contributing to elevated (higher than normal) triglycerides in the general population include: obesity and overweight, physical inactivity, cigarette smoking, excess alcohol intake, high carbohydrate diets (>60% of energy intake), several diseases (e.g., type 2 diabetes, chronic renal failure, nephrotic syndrome), certain drugs (e.g., corticosteroids, estrogens, retinoids, higher doses of beta-adrenergic blocking agents), and genetic disorders (familial combined hyperlipidemia, familial hypertriglyceridemia, and familial dysbetalipoproteinemia).

[ii] **Classification of Elevated Triglycerides**

In clinical practice, elevated serum triglycerides are most often observed in persons with the metabolic syndrome, although secondary or genetic factors can heighten triglyceride levels. ATP III adopts the following classification of serum triglycerides:

- Normal triglycerides: <150 mg/dL
- Borderline-high triglycerides: 150-199 mg/dL
- High triglycerides: 200-499 mg/dL
- Very high triglycerides: ≥500 mg/dL

[iii] **Non-HDL Cholesterol**

The finding that elevated triglycerides are an independent CHD risk factor suggests that some triglyceride-rich lipoproteins are atherogenic. The latter are partially degraded VLDL, commonly called *remnant lipoproteins.* In clinical practice, VLDL cholesterol is the most readily available measure of atherogenic remnant lipoproteins. Thus, VLDL cholesterol can be a target of cholesterol-lowering therapy. ATP III identifies the sum of LDL+VLDL cholesterol [termed *non-HDL cholesterol* (total cholesterol minus HDL cholesterol)] as a secondary target of therapy in persons with high triglycerides (≥200 mg/dL). The goal for non-HDL cholesterol in persons with high serum triglycerides can be set at 30 mg/dL higher than that for LDL cholesterol on the premise that a VLDL cholesterol level ≤30 mg/dL is normal.

[iv]   Association with LDL Cholesterol

Triglycerides cause the formation of the artherogenic, small, dense LDL particles. Four classes of LDL particles exhibit distinct biochemical and pathophysiological properties. (**TABLE**) Reduced LDL receptor binding is associated with the densest and the most buoyant, compared to the mid-density particles.

Particle	LDL-I	LDL-2	LDL-3	LDL-4
Predominant in Pattern	A	A	B	B

A normal pattern "A" consists of predominantly large, buoyant LDL species (LDL I-II). Pattern "B" consists of predominantly small, dense LDL (LDL III-IV), and is found in about 30-35% of adult men.[23] The density of the LDL particle is related to the triglyceride content. High triglyceride content of VLDL increases the transfer of triglycerides to LDL by the action of lipoprotein lipase, and increases the transfer of cholesterol to the remnant particle from the LDL. Buoyant, high triglyceride-containing LDL are subsequently metabolized by hepatic lipase to form the lipid-poor, dense LDL particles.

Lipoprotein pattern B phenotype, found in about 30% of the population is associated with an increased risk of CAD and non-insulin dependent diabetes mellitus, independent of age, smoking, gender, diabetes, HDL and LDL, but not plasma triglyceride.[24] Fifty percent of men with CAD have pattern B.[25] Only 17% of patients with pattern A phenotype have triglycerides above 95 mg/dL; whereas, only 17% of pattern B phenotype subjects have triglycerides below 95 mg/dL.[26] Pattern B can be converted to pattern A by lowering the triglyceride concentration with nicotinic acid.

[v]   Treatment

The treatment strategy for elevated triglycerides depends on the causes of the elevation and its severity. For all persons with elevated triglycerides, the primary aim of therapy is to achieve the target goal for LDL cholesterol. When triglycerides are *borderline high* (150-199 mg/dL), emphasis should also be placed on weight reduction and increased physical activity. For *high triglycerides* (200-499 mg/dL), non-HDL cholesterol becomes a secondary target of therapy. Aside from weight reduction and increased physical activity, drug therapy can be considered in high-risk persons to achieve the non- HDL cholesterol goal.

There are two approaches to drug therapy. First, the non-HDL cholesterol goal can be achieved by intensifying therapy with an LDL-lowering drug; or second, nicotinic acid or fibrate can be added, if used with appropriate caution, to achieve the non-HDL cholesterol goal by further lowering of VLDL cholesterol. In rare cases in which triglycerides are *very high* (≥ 500 mg/dL), the initial aim of therapy is to prevent acute pancreatitis through triglyceride lowering. This approach requires very low fat diets ($\leq 15\%$ of calorie intake), weight reduction, increased physical activity, and usually a triglyceride-lowering drug (fibrate or nicotinic acid). Only after triglyceride levels have been lowered to <500 mg/dL should attention turn to LDL lowering to reduce risk for CHD.

[c]   Low HDL Cholesterol

Low HDL cholesterol is a strong independent predictor of CHD. In ATP III, low HDL cholesterol is defined categorically as a level <40 mg/dL, a change from the level of <35 mg/dL in ATP II. In the present guidelines, low HDL cholesterol both modifies the goal for LDL-lowering therapy and is used as a risk factor to estimate 10-year risk for CHD.

Low HDL cholesterol levels have several causes, many of which are associated with insulin resistance, i.e., elevated triglycerides, overweight and obesity, physical inactivity, and type 2 diabetes. Other causes are cigarette smoking, very high carbohydrate intakes (>60% of calories), and certain drugs (e.g., beta-blockers, anabolic steroids, progestational agents).

ATP III does not specify a goal for raising HDL. Although clinical trial results suggest that raising HDL will reduce risk, the evidence is insufficient to specify a goal of therapy. Furthermore, currently available drugs do not robustly raise HDL cholesterol. Nonetheless, a low HDL should receive clinical attention and management according to the following sequence. In all persons with low HDL cholesterol, the primary target of therapy is LDL cholesterol; ATP III guidelines should be followed to achieve the LDL cholesterol goal. Second, after the LDL goal has been reached, emphasis shifts to weight reduction and increased physical activity (when the metabolic syndrome is present).

[i]   Low HDL with "Normal" LDL – LDL Particle Size

One of the most fascinating concepts to emerge from recent lipid research is that of LDL particle size. In brief, this concept explains how a person with low (or even normal) HDL and a normal LDL can still be at risk for cardiovascular disease. Conventional lipid tests measure the amount of cholesterol in the LDL fraction of the blood, not the particle size. Much research supports the concept that the smaller more dense LDL particles are more dangerous than the large buoyant LDL particles.[27]

One study indicated that the increased risk of CVD is not only affected by the levels of LDL in the blood, but the size of the LDL particles. Investigators found that increased amounts of small LDL particles were associated with a marked increase in the risk of CVD – even in the presence of

150

normal LDL levels. In other words, one person could have the same total LDL blood levels as another, but one could have a larger number of small LDL particles, placing that person at a higher cardiovascular risk (see below).[28]

Another study in the LDL particle size question investigated a group of people who characteristically have exceptional longevity and lower incidence of age-related disease. In comparing their blood and offspring's blood levels of HDL and LDL to other adults, investigators found the individuals with exceptional longevity had larger HDL and LDL particle sizes. These findings suggest that lipoprotein particle sizes are heritable and promote a healthy aging phenotype.[29]

What is the danger of small LDL particles? LDL particles contribute to arteriosclerosis by attacking the arterial wall. The smaller the particle size, the greater the number of particles required to carry any given amount of cholesterol, and vice versa. An excessive number of small LDL particles circulating in the blood promotes movement into the subendothelial space and formation of plaques. When the number is low, particle movement is reduced, resulting in decreased risk. Smaller particles may also be more susceptible to oxidation, and resultant oxidative damage.[30]

Prospective data from the Quebec Cardiovascular Study[31] indicate that elevated LDL particle numbers and small LDL size predict CHD risk better than LDL cholesterol. However, small LDL without an elevated number of LDL particles does not confer excess risk. Though conventional lipid profiles do not measure the size and number of LDL particles, there are several commercial assays that do.[32]

So, how do we reduce the number of small LDL particles in our systems? One way is to avoid the consumption of transfats (hydrogenated or partially hydrogenated vegetable oils, such as soy bean oil, corn oil, etc.). A study recently reported in the American Journal of Clinical Nutrition (AJCN) on the effects of trans-fats in the diet and cholesterol, produced some interesting results. Cholesterol in the blood of people was analyzed after consuming five experimental diets for 35-day periods. The diets consisted of fat from butter or four various degrees of trans-fats. This study found that the LDL cholesterol particles decreased significantly in size with increasing amounts of dietary trans-fat intake.[33]

Trans-fats are formed during the hydrogenation of vegetable oils – a process that changes oils into semi liquids or solid fats. Examples of trans-fat foods are deep fried foods, some pastries, margarine, donuts and French fries.

Interestingly, the AJCN trans-fat study also found that even though the butter diet (saturated fat) was associated with the highest blood LDL concentration, the LDL particles found were the largest. They also found that the subjects with the highest plasma triglyceride concentrations also had the smallest LDL peak particle size.

Dietary intake of fish oil has been reported to have the effect of changing LDL particle size. A recent study found that docosahexaenoic acid (DHA) supplementation significantly increased LDL particle size. Eicosapentaenoic acid (EPA) did not have the same effect but both EPA and DHA reduced blood levels of triglycerides. DHA and EPA are abundant in coldwater fish oils.[34]

A second recent study indicates niacin may also be beneficial in effecting a shift in LDL particles from the small dense particles to large benign particles.[35]

[ii]   Low HDL with Elevated Triglycerides

When a low HDL cholesterol is associated with high triglycerides (200-499 mg/dL), secondary priority goes to achieving the non-HDL cholesterol goal, as outlined before. Also, if triglycerides are <200 mg/dL (isolated low HDL cholesterol), drugs for HDL raising (fibrates or nicotinic acid) can be considered; however, treatment for isolated low HDL is mostly reserved for persons with CHD and CHD risk equivalents.

[d]   Diabetic Dyslipidemia

This disorder is essentially atherogenic dyslipidemia (high triglycerides, low HDL, and small dense LDL) in persons with type 2 diabetes. Although elevated triglycerides and/or low HDL cholesterol are common in persons with diabetes, clinical trial results support the identification of LDL cholesterol as the primary target of therapy, as it is in those without diabetes. Since diabetes is designated a CHD risk equivalent in ATP III, the LDL cholesterol goal of therapy for most persons with diabetes will be <100 mg/dL. Furthermore, when LDL cholesterol is ≥130 mg/dL, most persons with diabetes will require initiation of LDL-lowering drugs simultaneously with TLC to achieve the LDL goal. When LDL cholesterol levels are in the range of 100-129 mg/dL at baseline or on treatment, several therapeutic options are available: increasing intensity of LDL-lowering therapy, adding a drug to modify atherogenic dyslipidemia (fibrate or nicotinic acid), or intensifying control of other risk factors including hyperglycemia. When triglyceride levels are ≥200 mg/dL, non-HDL cholesterol becomes a secondary target of cholesterol-lowering therapy.

[E]   ATP III 2004 Update

In July 2004, the NCEP published a paper entitled Implications of Recent Clinical Trials for the National Cholesterol Education Program Adult Treatment Panel III Guidelines, which updates some elements of the Adult Treatment Panel III (ATP III) cholesterol guidelines released in 2001. The ATP III update has been endorsed by the National Heart, Lung, and Blood Institute, the American Heart Association, and the American College of Cardiology. Based on a review of five clinical trials of cholesterol-lowering statin treatment that were conducted since the release of ATP III, the update offers options for more intensive cholesterol-lowering treatment for people at high risk and moderately-high risk for a heart attack.

The ATP III update emphasizes that therapeutic lifestyle changes – low saturated fat and low cholesterol diet, physical activity, and weight control – remain the cornerstone of treatment for lowering cholesterol levels.

The modifications in the ATP III Update are as follows:[36]

[1]   High-risk Patients

Individuals who have coronary heart disease (CHD) or disease of the blood vessels to the brain or extremities, or diabetes, or multiple (2 or more) risk factors that give them a greater than 20 percent chance of having a heart attack within 10 years:

ATP III ("old recommendations")	UPDATE ("new recommendations")
The treatment goal for high risk patients is an LDL less than 100 mg/dL.	The overall goal for high-risk patients is still an LDL less than 100 mg/dL. There is a therapeutic option to set the goal at an LDL less than 70 mg/dL for very high-risk patients – those who have had a recent heart attack, or those who have cardiovascular disease combined with either diabetes, or severe or poorly controlled risk factors (such as continued smoking), or metabolic syndrome (a cluster of risk factors associated with obesity that includes high triglycerides and low HDL cholesterol).
Recommended consideration of cholesterol-lowering drug treatment in addition to lifestyle therapy for LDL cholesterol levels 130 mg/dL or higher in high-risk patients. Characterized drug treatment for LDL levels 100-129 mg/dL as optional, and not needed for LDL less than 100 mg/dL.	Recommends consideration of drug treatment in addition to lifestyle therapy for LDL levels 100 mg/dL or higher in high-risk patients, and characterizes drug treatment as optional for LDL less than 100 mg/dL.

[2]   Moderately High-risk Patients

Individuals who have multiple (2 or more) CHD risk factors together with a 10-20 percent risk for a heart attack within 10 years:

ATP III	UPDATE
The treatment goal is an LDL less than 130 mg/dL, and drug treatment is recommended if LDL is 130 mg/dL or higher.	The overall goal for moderately high-risk patients is still an LDL less than 130 mg/dL. There is a therapeutic option to set the treatment goal at an LDL less than 100 mg/dL, and to use drug treatment if LDL is 100-129 mg/dL.

[3]   High-risk and Moderately High-risk Patients

ATP III	UPDATE
Did not explicitly emphasize achieving a certain percentage lowering of LDL cholesterol.	Advises that the intensity of LDL-lowering drug treatment in high-risk and moderately high-risk patients be sufficient to achieve at least a 30 percent reduction in LDL levels.

[4]   Moderate Risk Patients

Those with 2 or more risk factors plus a less than 10 percent risk for heart attack within 10 years, or lower risk – those with 0-1 risk factor, the update does not modify the ATP III recommendations.

C-REACTIVE PROTEIN (CRP)

- **Parameters measured:**   hs-CRP (high sensitivity C-reactive protein, high sensitivity CRP)

- **The test in a "nutshell":**   A nonspecific measure of inflammation; elevations are thought to be associated with an increased risk of cardiovascular disease.

- **Normal values (expressed as relative increased risk of cardiovascular disease)**

RELATIVE RISK	HS-CRP LEVEL
Low	< 1.0 mg/L
Average	1.0 to 3.0 mg/L
High	> 3.0 mg/L

PANIC VALUES!!

hs-CRP > 3.5 mg/L

- **Results in a "nutshell":**

PARAMETER	IMPLICATIONS
hs-CRP	No current consensus exists on when to get tested; the test is most often done in conjuction with other tests that are ordered to assess risk of heart disease, such as lipid profiles.

- **Test details**

1. CRP is a biochemical by-product that rises in level rapidly following an inflammatory stimulus (e.g., acute MI). Hepatocytes produce CRP in response to elevated IL-6 levels that occur during the acute phase of inflammation. Endothelial tissue can produce low levels of CRP.

2. Although the sensitivity range of standard CRP assays (3-200+ mg/L) is adequate to evaluate clinically significant inflammatory processes, the tests are not precise enough to sense small changes in CRP levels associated with CV risk in apparently healthy individuals. As a result, a high-sensitivity CRP (hs-CRP) assay has been developed and is currently in use. The hs-CRP assays can detect low-grade inflammatory activity (as low as 0.15 mg/dL) within the vascular system, which helps predict the first or recurrent coronary events.

155

3. Though no direct correlation has yet been made regarding lowering of hs-CRP levels and patient outcome, certain drugs do lower hs-CRP levels. These include the combination of ezetimibe and simvastatin[37], atorvastatin (alone)[38] or combined with fish oil (but not fish oil alone)[39], and simvastatin (alone).[40]

4. The most recent consensus conference regarding use of inflammatory markers in cardiovascular disease concluded the following regarding use of hs-CRP:[41]

    > "Measurement of hs-CRP is an independent marker of risk and, in those judged at intermediate risk by global risk assessment (10 to 20% risk of CHD per 10 years), at the discretion of the physician, may help direct further evaluation and therapy in the primary prevention of CVD. The benefits of such therapy based on this strategy remain uncertain."

    Measurements should be done twice. Patients with high levels (i.e., greater than 10 mg/L) should be repeated and the patient examined for sources of infection or inflammation. The guidelines suggest 3 categories of C-reactive protein levels: less than 1 mg/L is "low"; 1–3 mg/L is "average"; and greater than 3 mg/L is "high." No specific recommendations regarding patient management based on C-reactive protein levels are stated.

5. At this point in time, there appears to be no scientific literature that directly and experimentally tests the hypothesis that measurement of C-reactive protein to assess CHD risk results in improved patient outcomes. However, many experts believe that hs-CRP has emerged as a powerful predictor of cardiovascular diseases, particularly of coronary heart disease (CHD).[42]

6. In addition to predicting future cardiovascular events, even in apparently healthy persons, hs-CRP is of predictive value in patients with acute coronary syndromes. hs-CRP concentrations >3 mg/L at admission are associated with an increased incidence of recurrent angina, coronary revascularization, MI, and cardiovascular death.[43]

7. hs-CRP elevations, though not specifically associated with LV ejection fraction, are also an independent negative prognosticator for patients with heart failure.[44]

CHAPTER 12 – OTHER TESTS

DRUG AND ALCOHOL SCREENING

There are numerous types of drug and alcohol screens that may be obtained, and for as many reasons. Only a few practical comments are made here.

- **Parameters measured:** Urine screens; blood alcohol levels; blood and urine toxicology screening.

- **The test in a "nutshell":** Consider blood alcohol as a medical test. Health care professionals have been warned against determining serum alcohol concentrations solely for "legal" reasons without informed consent, since doing so might be considered "assault and battery." The medical need to counsel a patient regarding drunk driving obviates any legal concerns with serum alcohol determinations, since the test result can be used to treat and advise the patient.

PANCREATIC TESTS

- **Parameters measured:** Amylase, lipase.

- **The test in a "nutshell":** Ordered to help in evaluation of abdominal pain (pancreatitis, bowel rupture).

- **Normal values**

TEST	ADULT NORMAL VALUE
Amylase (serum)	< 130 U/L
Lipase	< 160 U/L

PANIC VALUES!!

Amylase > 500 U/L

- **Results in a "nutshell":**

PARAMETER	IMPLICATIONS
Amylase (serum)	Nonspecific measurements often elevated by pancreatitis or pancreatic cancer. Salivary glands also rich in amylase – isozymes may be required. Persistent elevations may indicate pancreatic pseudocyst. The presence of amylase in peritoneal lavage fluid is highly suggestive of bowel rupture from trauma.
Lipase	More sensitive than amylase for pancreatitis.

- **Test details**

Amylase

1. **Increased in**: acute pancreatitis, pancreatic neoplasm, pancreas abscess, pancreas pseudocyst, ascites, macroamylasemia, perforated peptic ulcer, intestinal obstruction, intestinal infarction, acute cholecystitis, appendicitis, ruptured ectopic pregnancy, peritonitis, salivary gland inflammation, diabetic ketoacidosis, drug use (morphine, acute alcohol intoxication), lung cancer, esophageal cancer, ovarian cancer.

2. **Decreased in**: hepatic necrosis, advanced chronic pancreatitis

3. Serum/urine amylase ratio – sometimes this test is helpful if the diagnosis is not clear. The renal clearance of amylase can be related to the relatively constant clearance of creatinine. Thie is called the amylase:creatinine clearance ratio (ACCR) and is calculated as follows:

ACCR (%) = (Urine Amylase (U/L) x serum creatinine (umol/L)) x 100 ÷ (Serum Amylase (U/L) x urine creatinine (umol/L))

Timed urines are unnecessary and therefore either a random urine or 2-4 hour collection may be used. The normal ACCR is in the range 2-5%. In acute pancreatitis, tubular reabsorption of amylase and other proteins is reduced and ACCR is increased: Values > 8% are not uncommon. Elevated ACCR is also seen in burns, ketoacidosis, renal insufficiency, myeloma, light chain proteinuria, march hemoglobinuria and following extracorporeal circulation, large IV doses of corticosteroids, duodenal perforation and extra-peritoneal surgery. In macroamylasemia, ACCR is usually < 2%.

4. In patients presenting to the emergency department with acute abdominal pain a normal serum amylase concentration is not sufficiently sensitive to rule out the diagnosis of acute pancreatitis.[45] Similarly, a normal serum amylase level taken within three hours after blunt abdominal trauma does not eliminate the possibility of pancreatic injury. However, a

serum amylase determination more than three hours after trauma may be useful in detecting pancreatic injury.[46]

5. Elevated amylase levels in pleural fluid, especially when the pleural fluid/serum amylase ratio is > 1, strongly suggest a malignant effusion often due to carcinoma of the lung.

Lipase

1. Lipase is an enzyme secreted by the pancreas into the small intestines. It catalyzes the breakdown of triglycerides into fatty acids. As with amylase, lipase appears in the blood following damage to the pancreatic acinar cells.

2. Highly specific for pancreatic diseases, though other conditions may cause elevations.

3. **Increased in**: acute pancreatitis, perforated peptic ulcer, early pancreatic carcinoma, pancreatic duct obstruction.

4. **Decreased in**: acute pancreatitis (severe)

MICROBIOLOGY TESTS

■ **Parameters measured:**   Gram stains, cultures, antibiotic sensitivity testing

■ **The test in a "nutshell":**

> **Gram stain** – a chemical process performed on dried specimens place on a microscope slide designed to show the presence of bacteria. Gram positive bacteria stain purple; gram negative bacteria stain reddish-pink.
>
> **Cultures** – use of various types of culture media to attempt to grow infectious organisms from a variety of body fluids.
>
> **Antibiotic** sensitivity testing – tests that determine whether or not a particular organism is susceptible to a particular antibiotic; often done in conjunction with cultures; when a causative organism is identified, it is tested for sensitivity to a battery of commonly used antibiotics.

CANCER SCREENING TESTS

- **Prostate-specific antigen (prostate cancer; PSA)[47]**

1.   Prostate-specific antigen (PSA) is a protein produced by the cells of the prostate gland. The PSA test measures the level of PSA in the blood. Because PSA is produced by the body and can be used to detect disease, it is sometimes called a biological marker or tumor marker.

2.   It is normal for men to have low levels of PSA in their blood; however, prostate cancer or benign conditions can increase PSA levels. As men age, both benign prostate conditions and prostate cancer become more frequent. The most common benign prostate conditions are prostatitis (inflammation of the prostate) and benign prostatic hyperplasia (BPH) (enlargement of the prostate). There is no evidence that prostatitis or BPH cause cancer, but it is possible for a man to have one or both of these conditions and to develop prostate cancer as well.

3.   The FDA has approved the PSA test along with a digital rectal exam (DRE) to help detect prostate cancer in men age 50 and older. The FDA has also approved the PSA test to monitor patients with a history of prostate cancer to see if the cancer has recurred.

4.   Recommendations for screening vary. Some encourage yearly screening for men over age 50, and some advise men who are at a higher risk for prostate cancer to begin screening at age 40 or 45. Others caution against routine screening, while still others counsel men about the risks and benefits on an individual basis and encourage men to make personal decisions about screening. Currently, Medicare provides coverage for an annual PSA test for all men age 50 and older.

5.   PSA test results report the level of PSA detected in the blood. The test results are usually reported as nanograms of PSA per milliliter (ng/ml) of blood. In the past, most health care providers considered PSA values below 4.0 ng/ml as normal. However, recent research found prostate cancer in men with PSA levels below 4.0 ng/ml.[48] Many are now using the following ranges, with some variation:

- 0 to 2.5 ng/ml is low
- 2.6 to 10 ng/ml is slightly to moderately elevated
- 10 to 19.9 ng/ml is moderately elevated
- 20 ng/ml or more is significantly elevated

There is no specific normal or abnormal PSA level. However, the higher a man's PSA level, the more likely it is that cancer is present. But because various factors can cause PSA levels to fluctuate, one abnormal PSA test does not necessarily indicate a need for other diagnostic tests.

161

6. Detection does not always mean saving lives: Even though the PSA test can detect small tumors , finding a small tumor does not necessarily reduce a man's chance of dying from prostate cancer. PSA testing may identify very slow-growing tumors that are unlikely to threaten a man's life. Also, PSA testing may not help a man with a fast-growing or aggressive cancer that has already spread to other parts of his body before being detected.

7. False positive tests – false positive test results (also called false positives) occur when the PSA level is elevated but no cancer is actually present. False positives may lead to additional medical procedures that have potential risks and significant financial costs and can create anxiety for the patient and his family. Most men with an elevated PSA test turn out not to have cancer; only 25 to 30 percent of men who have a biopsy due to elevated PSA levels actually have prostate cancer.[49]

- **Carcinoembryonic antigen (CEA)** – breast, colon cancer.

1. Carcinoembryonic antigen (CEA) is a normal protein present in the fetus. Its' production normally stops before birth and CEA should not normally be detectable, except for very small amounts, in the blood of healthy adults. Normal adult levels = 3-5 ng/ml (depending on smoking status).

2. Some types of cancers, especially breast and colon tumors, lead to increased CEA levels in the blood. Other conditions can also increase the CEA level. These include:

   - Cigarette smoking
   - Other cancers (e.g., pancreas, lung, ovary)
   - Chronic obstructive pulmonary disease (COPD)
   - Cirrhosis
   - Crohn's disease
   - Pancreatitis
   - Renal failure
   - Peptic ulcer

3. CEA levels can be used in patients with documented cancer to:

   - Determine how widespread the tumor is
   - Monitor the effects of treatment
   - Determine whether the tumor has returned after successful treatment

4. Certain types of cancer treatments, such as hormone therapy for breast cancer , may actually cause the CEA level to go up. This elevation does not accurately reflect the state of the disease. It is sometimes referred to as a "flare response." Recognition that a rise in

162

CEA may be temporary and due to therapy is significant. If this possibility is not taken into account, the patient may be unnecessarily discouraged. Further, treatment that is actually effective may be stopped or changed prematurely.

5.   CEA is not used as a screening tool in healthy patients without signs or symptoms of disease. Many cancers do not produce CEA. A normal CEA level does *not* rule out the presence of cancer.

■   **BRC gene tests** – breast, ovarian cancer

1.   BRCA1 and BRCA2 are tumor suppressor genes that, when working properly, help repair damage to DNA (a process that also prevents tumor development). Mutations in both the BRCA1 and BRCA2 genes are characterized by predisposition to breast cancer and ovarian cancer as well as prostate cancer (BRCA1) and other cancers (BRCA2). It is estimated that 5% to 10% of all women with breast cancer may have a mutation of the genes BRCA1 and BRCA2.[50] Specific mutations of BRCA1 and BRCA2 are more common in women of Jewish ancestry.

2.   The estimated lifetime risk of developing breast cancer for women with BRCA1 and BRCA2 mutations is 40% to 85%. Carriers with a history of breast cancer have an increased risk of contralateral (on the other side) disease that may be as high as 5% per year.[51] Mutations in either gene also confer an increased risk of ovarian cancer. In addition, mutation carriers may be at increased risk of other primary cancers.[52] Male carriers of BRCA2 mutations are also at increased risk for breast cancer.[53]

3.   Both men and women may inherit and pass on BRCA1 or BRCA2 mutations.

4.   Women who test positive for BRCA1 or BRCA2 genetic mutations are at higher risk of developing breast cancer and may wish to consider preventive measures. These may include:

   •   Increased screening
   •   Chemoprevention (tamoxifen)
   •   Prophylactic mastectomy

5.   Prognosis for breast cancer survival depends upon the stage at which breast cancer is diagnosed and may not be different between individuals with BRCA1 or BRCA2 cancer-predisposing mutations and controls.

■ HER-2 gene tests

1. The HER-2 gene encodes the production of a cell surface receptor protein known as the HER-2 protein or receptor. Normal cells express a small amount of HER-2 protein on their plasma membranes in a tissue-specific pattern.

2. In tumor cells, errors in DNA replication may result in multiple copies of a gene on a single chromosome. This alteration is known as gene amplification. Amplification of the HER-2 gene leads to an overexpression of HER-2 protein, resulting in increased cell division and a higher rate of cell growth.

3. HER-2 gene amplification may also be associated with transformation of normal cells to cancer cells. The HER-2 gene is present in excess (amplified) in 25% of patients with breast cancer.[54] These individuals have a worse prognosis, but may be candidates for a new type of antibody therapy, trastuzumab (Herceptin®; see below).[55]

4. HER-2 protein overexpression correlates with several negative prognostic variables, including estrogen receptor-negative status and positive lymph nodes. HER-2 gene amplification was found to be highly correlated with shortened disease-free survival and shortened overall survival of node-positive patients.[56]

5. Testing for HER-2 status plays a key role in the management of metastatic breast cancer. Patients whose tumors overexpress HER-2 are candidates for a new anti-HER-2 therapy, trastuzumab (Herceptin®). This is a monoclonal antibody to the HER-2 receptor. Trastuzumab (Herceptin®) is FDA approved for first-line use in combination with paclitaxel (Taxol®; a newer chemotherpeutic drug) for the treatment of HER-2 protein overexpressing metastatic breast cancer in patients who have not received chemotherapy for their metastatic disease. Herceptin® as a single agent is indicated for the treatment of HER-2 protein overexpressing metastatic breast cancer in patients who have received one or more chemotherapy regimens for their metastatic disease.[57]

CHAPTER 13 – CASE STUDIES

CASE 1 – *Right lower quadrant pain*
CASE 2 – *Weakness and weight loss for one month*
CASE 3 – *Feeling "run down" for two months*
CASE 4 – *Three months of fatigue*
CASE 5 – *Diabetic on hemodialysis with weakness and fatigue*
CASE 6 – *Urinary frequency and burning*
CASE 7 – *Flank pain, shaking chills, and fever*
CASE 8 – *Nausea, vomiting, and jaundice*
CASE 9 – *Weakness, fatigue, and jaundice*
CASE 10 – *Two months of painless jaundice*
CASE 11 – *Epigastric pain, emaciation, jaundice*
CASE 12 – *Nausea, vomiting, weakness, and abdominal pain*
CASE 13 – *Leg cramps, weakness, and nausea on a hot day*
CASE 14 – *Post-operative patient with decreased responsiveness*
CASE 15 – *Diabetic with nausea, vomiting, and tachypnea*
CASE 16 – *Diabetic with epigastric pain and weakness*
CASE 17 – *Hyperactivity and hyperventilation*
CASE 18 – *Dialysis patient with weakness*
CASE 19 – *Nausea, vomiting, and diarrhea for three days*
CASE 20 – *Vehicle crash victim with no apparent injuries*
CASE 21 – *"Alcohol on breath," lethargic, and uncooperative*

Please note that there is some repetition of material, particularly in the discussions, from case to case. This is because I intend each case to stand alone and not to rely on others for it to be clear. First, read the clinical scenario – decide what lab studies you might want to see. Then look at the first set of lab results in the case study and take it from there . . . As you work the cases, I suggest you try to come up with the answers on your own first, prior to looking at what I've said. To make this easier, I've tried to keep the questions and their answers on separate pages whenever possible. Finally, I have only included relevant parts of the various lab tests – this is to allow you to focus specifically on the issue at hand. Enjoy!

CASE 1

25 year old male with right lower quadrant (RLQ) pain; started periumbilically 2 days ago. Has anorexia, temp of 101, decreased bowel sounds, and rebound tenderness in the right lower quadrant.

Camp Rothenberg Infirmary
Complete Blood Cell Count (CBC)

TEST	PATIENT	NORMAL
WBC X 10^3	12.5	5.0-10.0
%Band	10	1-3
%Seg	70	50-62
%Eosin	1	1-4
%Baso	0	0-1
%Mono	1	0-5
%Lymph	18	25-45

QUESTIONS

6. What are the lab findings?
7. What is the diagnosis?
8. What diagnosis does the clinical picture make you think about?
9. If the patient's WBC count was 8.0, instead of 12.0, would you change your mind?

ANSWERS

1. What are the lab findings?

The findings are an elevated WBC count (leukocytosis) with an increase in the percentage of segs (neutrophilia) and bands (bandemia or shift to the left), and a mild decrease in the numbers of lymphocytes (lymphopenia).

2. What is the diagnosis?

Trick question (sort of) – remember, people *not* tests, make diagnoses. There is no way, with the information that you have, to make a diagnosis. On the other hand, if you wanted to say that the findings are compatible with, but not diagnostic for, an acute infectious process, likely bacterial (increased WBC count with a left shift), I'd be the first to agree.

3. What diagnosis does the clinical picture make you think about?

Appendicitis is a likely possibility, though other intra-abdominal conditions (e.g., ruptured hollow viscus) should also be considered. Clinically, anorexia is common in appendicitis.

4. If the patient's WBC count was 8.0, instead of 12.0, would you change your mind?

The shift to the left (bandemia) and increased percentages of neutrophils suggests acute infection (usually bacterial), regardless of the total WBC. A common mistake is to fail to perform a differential count when the WBC is within normal limits. Without the differential here, and a WBC of only 8.0, the unwary provider may be tempted to be less impressed with the patient's clinical picture. Of course, at least to me, the clinical picture is impressive enough (regardless of the WBC) to consider surgical consultation.

CASE 2

40 year old female who complains of weakness and weight loss for one month; appetite is slightly decreased but no other GI symptoms.

Camp Rothenberg Infirmary
Complete Blood Cell Count (CBC)

TEST	PATIENT	NORMAL
WBC X 10^3	3.5	5.0-10.0
%Band	0	1-3
%Seg	30	50-62
%Eosin	1	1-4
%Baso	0	0-1
%Mono	10	0-5
%Lymph	59	25-45

QUESTIONS

1. What are the lab findings?
2. What are some potential causes of the above WBC picture?
3. If the diagnosis was infectious mononucleosis, what might be seen on examination of the peripheral blood smear?

168

ANSWERS

1.   What are the lab findings?

The WBC is low (leukopenia) with a preponderance of lymphocytes (lymphocytosis) and a slight excess of monocytes (monocytosis).

2.   What are some potential causes of the above WBC picture?

With a low total WBC, always think of a viral infection. The increase in lymphocytes is also compatible with this. Though the increase in monocytes is small, this entire picture is certainly compatible with, *but not diagnostic for*, infectious mononucleosis. Other tests (e.g., Monospot®), along with clinical findings (e.g., splenomegaly, swollen lymph nodes) are necessary to make a diagnosis. Other causes of a similar WBC picture include cancer (of any type), drug-induced bone marrow toxicity, or bone marrow recovery following chemotherapy.

3.   If the diagnosis was infectious mononucleosis, what might be seen on examination of the peripheral blood smear?

Mononucleosis, as well as several other viral infections, results in abnormally-appearing lymphocytes. Typically, these are larger than normal and the nuclei have more jagged edges than usual. When these cells are noted in the laboratory, they are reported as "atypical lymphocytes."

CASE 3

19 year old white female complains of feeling "run down" for the past two months. She has been jogging more than usual in preparation for an upcoming marathon.

Camp Rothenberg Infirmary
Complete Blood Cell Count (CBC)

PARAMETER	PATIENT	NORMAL RANGE
RBC X 10^6	4.16	4.5-5.5
Hb g/dl	10.5	M 14.0-17.4 F 12.0-16.0
Hct (%)	31.2	M 36-48 F 42-52
MCV (fl)	75	84-96
MCH pg	25.2	28-34
MCHC g/dl	33.6	32-36

QUESTIONS

1.   What are the lab findings?
2.   Regarding the RBC count, what general condition is present?
3.   Describe how you would further classify the above condition.
4.   What are possible causes of this condition in the above patient?

ANSWERS

1. What are the lab findings?

The RBC count (RBC), hemoglobin (Hb) and hematocrit (Hct) are all low, as are the MCV and the MCH.

2. Regarding the RBC count, what general condition is present?

The above findings suggest anemia (decreased numbers of RBCs). We can further classify the type of anemia present, as discussed in the next question.

3. Describe how you would further classify the above condition.

To classify anemias, we determine whether the cells are "ugly" or not – in other words, are they normal sized, too big, or too small? The easiest way to do this is to look at the MCV, a direct reflection of cell size. In this case, the MCV is less than normal, so the red cells are small. This is termed a microcytic anemia. Remember, at least metaphorically speaking, that when there is an abnormality in the hemoglobin, it "collapses," leading to smaller red cells. So, the patient has a microcytic anemia due to some type of hemoglobin abnormality.

4. What are possible causes of this condition in the above patient?

The two main causes of microcytic anemias are iron deficiency and thalassemia. Unless we have more information (e.g., family history, Mediterranean origin), thalassemia is difficult to rule in or out. This lady could have chronic blood loss (i.e., iron deficiency) from menstruation, poor diet, chronic hematuria secondary to jogging, GI blood loss due to non-steroidal anti-inflammatory drugs, or a combination of these factors. Serum iron levels would help establish the diagnosis. On the other hand, some clinicians simply start iron replacement therapy and observe the clinical response. If iron deficiency is present, the patient's reticulocyte count will start to increase significantly within 1-2 weeks.

CASE 4

42 year old white male complains of fatigue for the past 3 months. He had a total gastrectomy 4 months ago, following a motor vehicle accident (MVA).

Camp Rothenberg Infirmary
Complete Blood Cell Count (CBC)

PARAMETER	PATIENT	NORMAL RANGE
RBC X 10^6	2.8	4.5-5.5
Hb g/dl	10.3	M 14.0-17.4 F 12.0-16.0
Hct (%)	31	M 36-48 F 42-52
MCV (fl)	110	84-96
MCH pg	36.8	28-34
MCHC g/dl	33	32-36

QUESTIONS

1. What are the lab findings?
2. Regarding the RBC count, what general condition is present?
3. Describe how you would further classify the above condition.
4. What are possible causes of this condition in the above patient?

ANSWERS

1.   What are the lab findings?

The RBC count (RBC), hemoglobin (Hb) and hematocrit (Hct) are all low; the MCV and the MCH are elevated.

2.   Regarding the RBC count, what general condition is present?

The above findings suggest anemia (decreased numbers of RBCs). We can further classify the type of anemia present, as discussed in the next question.

3.   Describe how you would further classify the above condition.

To classify anemias, we determine whether the cells are "ugly" or not – in other words, are they normal sized, too big, or too small? The easiest way to do this is to look at the MCV, a direct reflection of cell size. In this case, the MCV is greater than normal, so the red cells are big. This is termed a macrocytic anemia. Remember, at least metaphorically speaking, that when there is an abnormality in the DNA, it fails to pack together properly, leading to larger red blood cells. Often the WBCs are also affected, since they also contain DNA (to be perfectly correct, mature RBCs do not contain nuclei; they are extruded at the reticulocyte stage). On the peripheral smear, WBCs appear larger than usual, with multilobed nuclei. This patient has a macrocytic anemia due to some type of DNA abnormality.

4.   What are possible causes of this condition in the above patient?

The two most common causes of macrocytic anemia are folate and/or vitamin B12 deficiency. Liver disease can also result in a similar picture. This patient recently had a gastrectomy. Remember that vitamin B12 is absorbed in the ileum but in order for proper absorption to occur, intrinsic factor (made in the stomach) is required. Following a total gastrectomy and no vitamin B12 supplementation, patients develop vitamin B12 deficiency. Generally, the previously healthy individual has sufficient B12 stores to last a few months. Only then do the signs and symptoms of macrocytic anemia occur. It is also possible that simple folic acid deficiency is the cause of this patient's anemia, rather than vitamin B12 deficiency, despite the suggestive clinical history. It would be prudent to measure serum levels of both prior to institution of therapy.

CASE 5

34 year old black female; insulin-requiring diabetic on hemodialysis for 2 years; complains of gradually increasing weakness and fatigue over the past 4 months.

Camp Rothenberg Infirmary
Complete Blood Cell Count (CBC)

PARAMETER	PATIENT	NORMAL RANGE
RBC X 10^6	3.18	4.5-5.5
Hb g/dl	9.3	M 14.0-17.4 F 12.0-16.0
Hct (%)	28	M 36-48 F 42-52
MCV (fl)	88	84-96
MCH pg	28.7	28-34
MCHC g/dl	33.2	32-36

QUESTIONS

1. What are the lab findings?
2. Regarding the RBC count, what general condition is present?
3. Describe how you would further classify the above condition.
4. What are possible causes of this condition in the above patient?

174

ANSWERS

1. What are the lab findings?

The RBC count (RBC), hemoglobin (Hb) and hematocrit (Hct) are all low; the MCV and the MCH are normal.

2. Regarding the RBC count, what general condition is present?

The above findings suggest anemia (decreased numbers of RBCs). We can further classify the type of anemia present, as discussed in the next question.

3. Describe how you would further classify the above condition.

To classify anemias, we determine whether the cells are "ugly" or not – in other words, are they normal sized, too big, or too small? The easiest way to do this is to look at the MCV, a direct reflection of cell size. In this case, the MCV is normal, so the red cells are normal in size. This is termed a normocytic anemia. Normal red cell size suggests that the "intrinsic machinery" of the cell is intact. However, the bone marrow simply isn't making enough of these *normal cells* to keep up with the demand – and the patient becomes anemic.

4. What are possible causes of this condition in the above patient?

The most common causes of normocytic anemia are chronic disease or acute bleeding. Based on the patient's history, acute bleeding is unlikely. The patient's history of diabetes and chronic renal failure (CRF) both qualify as chronic diseases that may cause normocytic anemia. In the case of CRF, regardless of the cause, the patient's failing kidneys don't produce enough erythropoietin to sustain normal bone marrow activity. As a result, the patient has a chronic low grade anemia. In fact, many clinicians refer to patients with CRF as being members of the "10/30 Club," meaning that their usual *baseline* Hb is around 10, and the Hct around 30. This fact can be very helpful in ongoing care and monitoring of renal failure patients.

Remember, there is a difference between *baseline* and *normal*. Patients with CRF are not expected to have normal values of H/H. Rather, when they are relatively stable (at their baseline), they run an H/H of 10/30. So, if you see a CRF patient whose H/H is significantly lower than 10/30 (i.e., 7/21), don't attribute the anemia to CRF alone. This is *way below* the average for renal failure patients and suggests an additional cause, usually bleeding.

CASE 6

29 year old female complains of 1 day of urinary frequency, burning, and reddish staining of her underwear. She has no back pain, nausea, or vomiting. The patient appears well-hydrated; normal vital signs present.

Camp Rothenberg Infirmary
Urinalysis (UA)

PARAMETER	PATIENT RESULT	NORMAL RANGE
Color	Yellow	Pale yellow to amber
Appearance	Cloudy	Clear to slightly hazy
Specific gravity	1.020	1.015-1.025
pH	6.0	4.5-8.0
Glucose	-	Negative
Ketones	-	Negative
Blood	+++	Negative
Protein	-	Negative
Bilirubin	-	Negative
Urobilinogen	tr	Negative-trace
Nitrate for bacteria	++	Negative
Leucocyte esterase	+++	Negative
Casts	-	Negative
RBC	+++	Rare or negative
WBC	++	Negative or rare
Crystals	-	Negative
Epithelial cells	+	Few
Bacteria	+++	None

QUESTIONS

1. What are the lab findings?
2. Based on the clinical picture, what conditions are possible?
3. Does the patient look "sick" or "not sick" clinically?
4. Based on the above information, what is the most likely working diagnosis?

176

5. **Is a urine culture and sensitivity (C&S) necessary at this point?**

ANSWERS

1. **What are the lab findings?**

The urine is cloudy and the dipstick is positive for blood, nitrite, and leukocyte esterase. On microscopic examination, no casts are present. However, numerous red and white cells, as well as bacteria are seen.

2. **Based on the clinical picture, what conditions are possible?**

Clinically, the patient's presentation is compatible with an uncomplicated, lower urinary tract infection (UTI). It is possible, however, that she may have a low-grade upper tract infection (pyelonephritis) or even a vaginal infection.

3. **Does the patient look "sick" or "not sick" clinically?**

The patient does not look "sick." This is an important determination to make early on. Even if the working diagnosis turns out to be a potentially more serious condition, such as pyelonephritis, stable patients who are not pregnant and are not diabetic can often be treated as outpatients.

4. **Based on the above information, what is the most likely working diagnosis?**

The urine is compatible with UTI – if casts would have been present, involvement of the upper urinary tract would have been implicated (i.e., pyelonephritis). Their absence, however, does *not* exclude pyelonephritis but the clinical picture makes it less likely (absence of back pain, nausea, vomiting; patient not "sick"). Though we'd have to perform a pelvic examination to completely exclude some type of vaginal infection, the patient's symptoms fit UTI far better. I'm going to bet on an uncomplicated UTI and treat her with an oral antibiotic and antispasmodic.

5. **Is a urine culture and sensitivity (C&S) necessary at this point?**

Most common organisms are susceptible to common antibiotics, such as trimethoprim-sulfamethoxazole (Septra®, Bactrim®) or amoxicillin. Many clinicians would simply treat this patient empirically, both with an antibiotic *and* an antispasmodic (e.g., phenazopyridine [Pyridium®]). If her symptoms did not clear up within 48 hours, a urine C&S would be warranted.

CASE 7

35 year old male complains of two days of bilateral flank pain, shaking chills, fever. He's also had nausea and vomiting for 1 day and a decreased appetite. Patient's temperature is 102.5° F. His tongue is furrowed and there is 1+ tenting of the arm skin.

Camp Rothenberg Infirmary
Urinalysis (UA)

PARAMETER	PATIENT RESULT	NORMAL RANGE
Color	Dk yellow	Pale yellow to amber
Appearance	Turbid	Clear to slightly hazy
Specific gravity	1.026	1.015-1.025
pH	5.0	4.5-8.0
Glucose	-	Negative
Ketones	-	Negative
Blood	++	Negative
Protein	+	Negative
Bilirubin	-	Negative
Urobilinogen	tr	Negative-trace
Nitrate for bacteria	+++	Negative
Leucocyte esterase	+++	Negative
Casts	WBC, RBC	Negative
RBC	++	Rare or negative
WBC	+++	Negative or rare
Crystals	-	Negative
Epithelial cells	few	Few
Bacteria	+	None

QUESTIONS

1.   What are the lab findings?
2.   Based on the clinical picture, what conditions are possible?
3.   Does the patient look "sick" or "not sick" clinically?
4.   Based on the above information, what is the most likely working diagnosis?

5.   **Is a urine culture and sensitivity (C&S) necessary at this point?**

ANSWERS

1.   **What are the lab findings?**

The urine is turbid and the dipstick is positive for blood, nitrite, and leukocyte esterase. On microscopic examination, both RBC and WBC casts are present. Numerous red and white cells, as well as bacteria are seen.

2.   **Based on the clinical picture, what conditions are possible?**

This patient's clinical presentation is strongly suggestive of acute pyelonephritis. An uncomplicated UTI should not cause significant fever or nausea and vomiting. A person's appetite is not usually affected, either. It is always possible that some other type of febrile illness, even a moderately severe viral syndrome (the "flu") could result in a similar picture, but we'd better consider pyelonephritis first.

3.   **Does the patient look "sick" or "not sick" clinically?**

The patient is moderately dehydrated (tongue furrowing, tenting of the skin, urine specific gravity slightly elevated), and certainly appears uncomfortable. Even if the vital signs, other than temperature, are normal, I'd classify him as "sick."

4.   **Based on the above information, what is the most likely working diagnosis?**

The clinical picture, combined with the UA (especially the presence of WBC and RBC casts) is most compatible with acute pyelonephritis and moderate dehydration. Patients who are "sick" like this need to be hospitalized for both intravenous fluids and antibiotics, at least for 24-48 hours.

5.   **Is a urine culture and sensitivity (C&S) necessary at this point?**

Though most clinicians would start empiric antibiotics (often a cephalosporin), most would also obtain a urine C&S to make certain their choice was appropriate. I'd also get a couple of sets of blood cultures. Bacteremia can develop in up to 30% of patients with pyelonephritis, sometimes leading to full-blown sepsis syndrome. The earlier bacteremia is discovered, the more aggressive the clinician can be in an attempt to prevent sepsis.

CASE 8

17 year old white male who visited with friends out of town for a week. About a month later, he developed weakness, nausea, intermittent vomiting, and a change in the color of his urine. He is moderately tender in the right upper quadrant and has 2+ scleral icterus.

Camp Rothenberg Infirmary
Urinalysis (UA)

PARAMETER	PATIENT RESULT	NORMAL RANGE
Color	orange-yellow	Pale yellow to amber
Appearance	clear	Clear to slightly hazy
Specific gravity	1.020	1.015-1.025
pH	5.0	4.5-8.0
Glucose	-	Negative
Ketones	-	Negative
Blood	-	Negative
Protein	-	Negative
Bilirubin	+++	Negative
Urobilinogen	tr	Negative -trace
Nitrate for bacteria	-	Negative
Leucocyte esterase	-	Negative
Casts	-	Negative
RBC	-	Rare or negative
WBC	-	Negative or rare
Crystals	-	Negative
Epithelial cells	-	Few
Bacteria	-	None

QUESTIONS

1. What are the lab findings?
2. Mechanistically, what do these suggest regarding the hepatobiliary system?
3. What additional lab tests do you want to obtain?

ANSWERS

1.   What are the lab findings?

The urine is an abnormal orange color. Though the microscopic examination is completely negative, the dipstick is abnormal – 3+ bilirubin is present in the urine. The trace of urobilinogen is normal.

2.   Mechanistically, what do these suggest regarding the hepatobiliary system?

Remember, when you see a "yellow fellow," give 'em a cup and do a "dip UA." The presence of bilirubin in the urine is always abnormal – to appear in the urine, bilirubin must first be conjugated (water-soluble). In addition, bilirubin in the urine must never have gotten to the bowel in the first place – if it did, it would be converted into urobilinogen and be passed in either the feces (as "brown dye #2") or in the urine (as urinary urobilinogen). As we've said earlier, bilirubinuria indicates some type of liver or biliary drainage system problem – hepatobiliary disease. There are only two generic mechanisms whereby bilirubin can 1) be conjugated and 2) *not* pass into the bowel:

- Failure of hepatic secretion – hepatocellular injury (e.g., hepatitis, toxin) damages the hepatocytes such that *some* of this process is lost – a portion of conjugated bilirubin cannot be passed into the bile canaliculi and then into the bile. As a result, it backs up into the blood, often causing clinical jaundice. Since this bilirubin is water-soluble, it is filtered in the kidney and passes out of the body in the urine.

- Obstruction (either partial or complete) – conjugated bilirubin is secreted into the biliary drainage tree but can't get to the bowel due to some type of a blockage. Sometimes, this takes place in the liver (e.g., primary biliary cirrhosis). Other times, the obstruction is outside of the liver (e.g., pancreatic cancer). Either way, bilirubin that doesn't pass into the gut can't be converted into urobilinogen, right? So if there's complete obstruction, it's impossible to have any urobilinogen in the urine. The bilirubin that can't make it to the bowel due to obstruction will back up into the blood. As detailed above, it then passes out of the body in the urine.

The fact that our patient has a small amount of urobilinogen in his urine effectively rules out complete biliary obstruction. So, his problem is either due to *partial* obstruction or failure of hepatic secretion (hepatocellular injury). Combined with the clinical picture you already have, we'll use additional tests and information in just a little bit to decide which is more likely.

3.   What additional lab tests do you want to obtain?

For now, let's go with a CBC and a Liver Panel.

181

Camp Rothenberg Infirmary
Complete Blood Cell Count (CBC)

PARAMETER	PATIENT RESULT	NORMAL RANGE
WBC X 10^3	4.5	5.0-10.0
%Band	0	1-3
%Seg	15	50-62
%Eosin	1	1-4
%Baso	1	0-1
%Mono	5	0-5
%Lymph	78	25-45
RBC X 10^6	nl	4.5-5.5
Hb g/dl	nl	M 14.0-17.4 F 12.0-16.0
Hct (%)	nl	M 36-48 F 42-52
MCV (fl)	nl	84-96
MCH pg	nl	28-34
MCHC g/dl	nl	32-36
Plts X 10^3	nl	140-400

QUESTIONS

1. What are the lab findings?
2. What are some potential causes of the above WBC picture?
3. With the information you have so far, what diagnostic possibilities seem most likely?
4. What is the next step in narrowing down the diagnosis?

ANSWERS

1. **What are the lab findings?**

The CBC shows a low total WBC (leukopenia) with a significant decrease in the percentage of neutrophils (neutropenia), and a significant increase in the percentage of lymphocytes (lymphocytosis). The red blood cells and platelets are WNL.

2. **What are some potential causes of the above WBC picture?**

Leukopenia with lymphocytosis suggests, but does not prove, a viral infection. Another possible explanation is bone marrow suppression due to any cause. A potentially bothersome finding is that the total number of neutrophils is significantly decreased – 15% of 4500 = 675 total neutrophils. Increased susceptibility to bacterial infections starts to become an issue when the total neutrophil count falls below 1000, however, the risk is greatest when the number is below 500 cells. Realistically, this is probably not a concern in this patient as long as he was previously healthy.

3. **With the information you have so far, what diagnostic possibilities seem most likely?**

The lab picture so far suggests some type of hepatobiliary disease (bilirubinuria) without complete obstruction (urobilinogen present in the urine), as well as a viral infection (leukopenia with lymphocytosis). The two most likely diagnostic possibilities at this point are viral hepatitis or infectious mononucleosis (which often causes a hepatitis-like picture, especially if due to cytomegalovirus [CMV]). Primary biliary cirrhosis, tumor, or other form of partial biliary obstruction seem unlikely in light of the clinical history.

4. **What is the next step in narrowing down the diagnosis?**

Looking at the liver profile for evidence of hepatocellular injury (increased ALT/AST [SGPT/SGOT]) is necessary at this point to confirm the above suspicions.

Camp Rothenberg Infirmary
Liver Panel

Parameter	Patient result	Normal value (adults)
Bilirubin, total	2.8	0.2-1.0 mg/dl
Bilirubin, direct (conjugated)	2.4	0.0-0.2 mg/dl
Bilirubin, indirect (unconjugated)	.4	0.2-0.8 mg/dl
Alanine transaminase (ALT, SGPT [serum glutamic-pyruvic transaminase])	250	7-56 U/L
Alkaline phosphatase (ALP)	250	17-142 IU/L
Aspartate transaminase (AST; serum glutamic-oxaloacetic transaminase [SGOT])	800	5-40 U/L

QUESTIONS

1. What are the lab findings?
2. What diagnostic category of jaundice do they suggest?
3. Which clinical diagnoses are compatible with the findings (clinical and lab) so far?
4. What additional laboratory tests could you perform to further narrow down the diagnosis?

ANSWERS

1. What are the lab findings?

The liver panel shows elevated total bilirubin, mostly conjugated, increased alkaline phosphatase, and increased liver enzyme levels (ALT/AST, SGPT/SGOT).

2. What diagnostic category of jaundice do they suggest?

Elevations of alkaline phosphatase in a 17-year old are difficult to interpret. They could be present simply because his bones are still growing and the epiphyses have yet to close. Hepatocellular or obstructive hepatobiliary disease could also lead to raised alkaline phosphatase levels since the enzyme is excreted in a fashion similar to bilirubin (into the hepatobiliary drainage tree, then into the bowel).

Elevation of the total bilirubin is not surprising, in light of the fact that the patient is clinically jaundiced. Remember, the presence of clinical jaundice indicates that the total bilirubin level is at least 2-3 times normal, as a rule. And, since there is bilirubinuria, the majority of the bilirubin elevation is due to excess of the conjugated form.

Obstruction, either partial or complete, does not usually result in an increase in the liver enzymes. Elevations of ALT/AST (SGPT/SGOT) greater than two times normal, as is the care here, suggest hepatocellular injury (e.g., hepatitis, toxin).

3. Which clinical diagnoses are compatible with the findings (clinical and lab) so far?

Viral hepatitis is the most likely diagnosis, based on the information currently available. Infectious mononucleosis is also a diagnostic possibility. Other forms of hepatitis, such as alcoholic hepatitis, may have similar laboratory features and would have to be excluded on the basis of history.

4. What additional laboratory tests could you perform to further narrow down the diagnosis?

A Monospot® test, Ebstein-Barr virus or CMV antibodies would help in the diagnosis of infectious mononucleosis. If viral hepatitis is suspected, a variety of tests should be obtained (see section on Hepatitis Tests, Chapter 6).

CASE 9

24 year old female started on sulfamethoxazole-trimethoprim (Septra, Bactrim) for a UTI. Now complains of weakness, fatigue, and bloody urine. She has no chills, fever, anorexia, nausea, or vomiting. She has 1+ scleral icterus.

Camp Rothenberg Infirmary
Urinalysis (UA)

PARAMETER	PATIENT RESULT	NORMAL RANGE
Color	yellow	Pale yellow to amber
Appearance	clear	Clear to slightly hazy
Specific gravity	1.021	1.015-1.025
pH	7.0	4.5-8.0
Glucose	-	Negative
Ketones	-	Negative
Blood	-	Negative
Protein	-	Negative
Bilirubin	-	Negative
Urobilinogen	+++	Negative-trace
Nitrate for bacteria	-	Negative
Leucocyte esterase	-	Negative
Casts	-	Negative
RBC	-	Rare or negative
WBC	-	Negative or rare
Crystals	-	Negative
Epithelial cells	-	Few
Bacteria	-	None

QUESTIONS

1.   What are the lab findings?
2.   Mechanistically, what do these suggest regarding the hepatobiliary system?
3.   What additional lab tests do you want to obtain?

ANSWERS

1. What are the lab findings?

The only abnormality on the UA is a significant increase in urinary urobilinogen levels. No bilirubin is present.

2. Mechanistically, what do these suggest regarding the hepatobiliary system?

The absence of bilirubinuria in a jaundiced patient suggests that the cause of his or her jaundice is *not* related to hepatobiliary system disease. Only conjugated bilirubin can appear in the urine. Thus, a jaundiced patient without bilirubinuria must have an excess of unconjugated (albumin-bound, nonwater soluble) bilirubin in the blood. Mechanistically, there are two basic causes:

- Overload of hemoglobin for the liver to metabolize – this occurs in the face of either a hemolytic anemia or reabsorption of a large hematoma. Either way, the amount of hemoglobin that the "mortuary" (spleen) needs to metabolize is increased significantly. As a result, more indirect bilirubin is sent to the liver for conjugation. The liver enzyme systems can only move so fast; thus, indirect (albumin-bound) bilirubin backs up in the blood, causing jaundice, until it can be conjugated. Once conjugated, the bilirubin follows the normal excretory pathways.

  The only difference between normal bilirubin metabolism and hemolysis or hematoma reabsorption is that *more* conjugated bilirubin is produced – this is a necessary result of the "law of mass action." This law states: "More in, more out." If more indirect bilirubin is put through the liver conjugation process (because of excessive red cell death), more conjugated bilirubin must be produced. And, when this conjugated bilirubin goes to the bowel, *more* urobilinogen must be produced. Only so much urobilinogen goes out in the stool. The rest passes in the urine. Since there is more urobilinogen made in the bowel under these circumstances, it stands to reason that there will be *more* to pass out in the urine. In this type of jaundice, urinary urobilinogen levels rise, indicating production of excess urobilinogen in the bowel. Since all the bilirubin eventually makes it to the bowel, it is converted to urobilinogen and no bilirubin appears in the urine.

- Conjugation defect – conjugation defects are deficiencies in the liver enzymes that normally catalyze the conjugation of bilirubin. The two most common types are neonatal jaundice and, in adults, Gilbert's Syndrome. In a conjugation defect, the normal amount of unconjugated bilirubin is presented to the liver for conjugation. Since the enzyme systems move "slower than usual," conjugation takes place at a slower rate. So, unconjugated bilirubin (albumin-bound) backs up in the serum, waiting to be conjugated. The result is jaundice.
  Eventually, the indirect bilirubin is conjugated, especially if the enzyme deficiency

187

is transient (which is common in both neonatal jaundice and in Gilbert's syndrome). Since there was no additional indirect bilirubin sent to the liver for conjugation, the total amount of bilirubin conjugated is *not* increased. And, there is no increase in urobilinogen production in the bowel. So, it's unlikely that there will be much excess urobilinogen present that didn't pass out with the stool. As a result, in conjugation defects the urine urobilinogen is *not* elevated (remember, normal = negative to trace). And, since it's all converted to urobilinogen, no conjugated bilirubin passes out in the urine (the dipstick is negative for bilirubin).

3.　　**What additional lab tests do you want to obtain?**

If hemolytic anemia is a possibility, checking a CBC would be helpful. Some would also order a Liver Panel at this point, though the results in many cases don't tell you anything that you didn't already know (read on . . .).

Camp Rothenberg Infirmary
Complete Blood Cell Count (CBC)

PARAMETER	PATIENT RESULT	NORMAL RANGE
WBC X 10^3	8.5	5.0-10.0
%Band	1	1-3
%Seg	55	50-62
%Eosin	1	1-4
%Baso	1	0-1
%Mono	3	0-5
%Lymph	39	25-45
RBC X 10^6	3.41	4.5-5.5
Hb g/dl	9.8	M 14.0-17.4 F 12.0-16.0
Hct (%)	29.4	M 36-48 F 42-52
MCV (fl)	86	84-96
MCH pg	28.7	28-34
MCHC g/dl	33	32-36
Plts X 10^3	150	140-400

QUESTIONS

1. What are the lab findings?
2. Regarding the RBC count, what general condition is present?
3. Describe how you would further classify the above condition.
4. What are possible causes of this condition in the above patient?
5. What would you expect to see on the Liver Panel?

189

ANSWERS

1. **What are the lab findings?**

   The RBC count (RBC), hemoglobin (Hb) and hematocrit (Hct) are all low; the MCV and the MCH are normal. WBCs and platelet counts are normal.

2. **Regarding the RBC count, what general condition is present?**

   The above findings suggest anemia (decreased numbers of RBCs). We can further classify the type of anemia present, as discussed in the next question.

3. **Describe how you would further classify the above condition.**

   To classify anemias, we determine whether the cells are "ugly" or not – in other words, are they normal sized, too big, or too small? The easiest way to do this is to look at the MCV, a direct reflection of cell size. In this case, the MCV is normal, so the red cells are normal in size. This is termed a normocytic anemia. Normal red cell size suggests that the "intrinsic machinery" of the cell is intact. However, the bone marrow simply isn't making enough of these *normal cells* to keep up with the demand – and the patient becomes anemic.

4. **What are possible causes of this condition in the above patient?**

   The most common causes of normocytic anemia are chronic disease or acute bleeding. The patient has no history of chronic disease to explain the normocytic anemia. Similarly, there is no history of acute external bleeding (e.g., secondary to trauma). On the other hand, hemolytic anemia is a form of internal bleeding, at least as far as it affects the CBC. RBCs are lost, leading to decreased H/H, but those cells and the nonhemolyzed RBCs are normal – resulting in a normal MCV and a normocytic anemia. An increase in the patient's urinary urobilinogen is also compatible with acute hemolytic anemia.

   If the above patient has a hemolytic anemia, her recently prescribed sulfa drugs are the most likely cause. This is an uncommon, but well-described side effect of these drugs, especially in a person with previously unknown X-linked recessive congenital deficiency of the enzyme G6PD (glucose-6-phosphate dehydrogenase; the most common human enzyme deficiency – an estimated 400 million people worldwide are affected). Persons with G6PD deficiency are unable to break down free radicals produced during the metabolism of certain drugs (e.g., sulfa drugs). As a result, the free radicals attack RBC membranes, leading to intravascular hemolysis. Of course, it's always possible that the patient has an acquired autoimmune hemolytic anemia from another cause, such as lupus.

190

The list of medications that persons with known G6PD deficiency should avoid is extensive. For further information on this topic, including a long list of medications patients should avoid, see: http://rialto.com/g6pd/ (great site!!).

5.   **What would you expect to see on the Liver Panel?**

Since the patient is clinically jaundiced, the total bilirubin should be elevated. The unconjugated fraction should be higher, since there is no bilirubinuria. I'd expect alkaline phosphatase, ALT (SGPT), and AST (SGOT) levels to all be normal, since hemolytic anemia is *not* an intrinsic disease of the hepatobiliary system. Let's take a look . . .

Camp Rothenberg Infirmary
Liver Panel

Parameter	Patient result	Normal value (adults)
Bilirubin, total	4.5	0.2-1.0 mg/dl
Bilirubin, direct (conjugated)	0.5	0.0-0.2 mg/dl
Bilirubin, indirect (unconjugated)	4.0	0.2-0.8 mg/dl
Alanine transaminase (ALT, SGPT [serum glutamic-pyruvic transaminase])	20	7-56 U/L
Alkaline phosphatase (ALP)	35	17-142 IU/L
Aspartate transaminase (AST; serum glutamic-oxaloacetic transaminase [SGOT])	26	5-40 U/L
Lactic acid dehydrogenase (LDH)	650	313-618 U/L

QUESTIONS

1. What are the lab findings?
2. Are they compatible with the presumptive diagnoses discussed above?
3. What other tests might you consider obtaining?

ANSWERS

1. What are the lab findings?

The total bilirubin is elevated, as predicted in the face of clinical jaundice. The elevation consists mostly of unconjugated (albumin-bound) bilirubin – this makes sense, considering the lack of bilirubin in the urine. Enzymes (alkaline phosphatase, ALT/AST [SGPT/SGOT]) are normal.

2. Are they compatible with the presumptive diagnoses discussed above?

The above findings are compatible with, but not diagnostic for, hemolytic anemia. We expect to see an excess of unconjugated bilirubin (eventually leading to increased urobilinogen in the urine) and otherwise, relatively normal liver function tests (since the problem does not lie in the hepatobiliary system in the first place!).

Note that the total LDH value is elevated. Sometimes, this test is obtained as part of a Liver Panel. LDH isozymes 1 and 2 are found in RBCs, as well as in heart muscle (see text). Normally, the amount of LDH2 is greater than that of LDH1 (i.e., LDH2 > LDH1). In myocardial infarction and in hemolytic anemia LDH is released into the serum by damaged cells. For unknown reasons, the amount of LDH1 increases *more* than the amount of LDH2. The result is an increase in total LDH, as well as what is termed an LDH "flip," where LDH1 becomes greater than LDH2 (LDH1 > LDH2). LDH isozymes are not obtained routinely in the diagnosis of hemolytic anemia, but may be helpful if the picture is unclear.

3. What other tests might you consider obtaining?

Hemolytic anemia may occur due to chemical toxicity (as in G6PD deficiency) or due to the presence of antibodies (e.g., autoimmune hemolytic anemia). The following tests may be of additional assistance:

- Serum haptoglobin – decreased levels of haptoglobin are a sensitive indicator of hemolysis. Haptoglobin is a protein manufactured by the liver and secreted into the blood to bind free hemoglobin. Normally, blood free hemoglobin levels are very low, but with hemolysis, the amount increases considerably. After haptoglobin binds free hemoglobin, the complex is taken up by the liver and metabolized, breaking down both hemoglobin and haptoglobin. During hemolysis, the rate of haptoglobin destruction will outpace the rate at which new haptoglobin is created. As a result, the blood haptoglobin level decreases.

- Direct antiglobulin test (direct Coombs test) – a test for antibodies attached to the surface of red blood cells; positive in autoimmune hemolytic anemia, as well as in a number of other conditions: drug-induced hemolytic anemia, erythroblastosis fetalis (hemolytic disease of the newborn), infectious mononucleosis, mycoplasmal infection, syphilis, chronic lymphocytic leukemia, systemic lupus erythematosus and rheumatologic conditions, and transfusion reactions. Sometimes, this test is abnormal in apparently healthy people for no obvious reason – up to 3% of hospitalized patients with no known underlying condition have a positive direct antiglobulin test.

- Indirect antiglobulin test (indirect Coombs test) – tests for antibodies to RBCs in the blood; may indicate autoimmune hemolytic anemia or drug-induced hemolytic anemia.

- G6PD screen – can detect an enzyme deficiency unless the reticulocyte count is significantly elevated (reticulocytes contain a lot of G6PD).

- RBC survival (chromium Cr 51 survival) – a nuclear medicine test that determines the mean RBC life span (should normally be ~ 120 days). This test is not done commonly, but may help evaluate an unexplained anemia, especially when hemolysis is suspected. Occasionally used to test survival of transfused red cells in face of major problems in compatibility testing. The test is burdensome, requiring regular collection of specimens for up to four weeks.

CASE 10

42 year old female with painless jaundice, progressive over the past 2 months. She has no weakness, weight loss, nausea, or vomiting. She had a laparoscopic cholecystectomy 8 months ago in another city.

Camp Rothenberg Infirmary
Urinalysis (UA)

PARAMETER	PATIENT RESULT	NORMAL RANGE
Color	orange-red	Pale yellow to amber
Appearance	clear	Clear to slightly hazy
Specific gravity	1.020	1.015-1.025
pH	5.70	4.5-8.0
Glucose	-	Negative
Ketones	-	Negative
Blood	-	Negative
Protein	-	Negative
Bilirubin	+++	Negative
Urobilinogen	-	Negative-trace
Nitrate for bacteria	-	Negative
Leucocyte esterase	-	Negative
Casts	-	Negative
RBC	-	Rare or negative
WBC	-	Negative or rare
Crystals	-	Negative
Epithelial cells	-	Few
Bacteria	-	None

QUESTIONS

1. What are the lab findings?
2. Mechanistically, what do these suggest regarding the hepatobiliary system?
3. What additional lab tests do you want to obtain?

195

ANSWERS

1. **What are the lab findings?**

   The UA demonstrates two abnormalities – abnormal color (orange-red) and 3+ bilirubinuria. Note that no urobilinogen is present in the urine.

2. **Mechanistically, what do these suggest regarding the hepatobiliary system?**

   Remember, when you see a "yellow fellow," give 'em a cup and do a "dip UA." The presence of bilirubin in the urine is always abnormal – to appear in the urine, bilirubin must first be conjugated (water-soluble). In addition, bilirubin in the urine must never have gotten to the bowel in the first place – if it did, it would be converted into urobilinogen and be passed in either the feces (as "brown dye #2") or in the urine (as urinary urobilinogen). As we've said earlier, bilirubinuria indicates some type of liver or biliary drainage system problem – hepatobiliary disease. There are only two generic mechanisms whereby bilirubin can 1) be conjugated and 2) *not* pass into the bowel (see Case 8) – failure of hepatic secretion (e.g., hepatitis, toxin) or obstruction (complete or partial).

   In this case, our patient has painless jaundice, large amounts of bilirubin in the urine, and no detectable urobilinogen. The combination is worrisome and, until proven otherwise, indicates complete obstruction somewhere in the hepatobiliary drainage system. If complete obstruction is present, there is no way for bilirubin to get into the bowel. As a result, no urobilinogen can be made. Remember that urobilinogen, reacting with stool in formation, causes the brown color of stool. So, though it's not mentioned in the above information, I wouldn't be surprised if the patient had acholic (clay-colored stools). No brown dye #2, no brown stool – right?

3. **What additional lab tests do you want to obtain?**

   My personal opinion is that there are no lab tests that will change my mind at this point – the patient needs a CT scan, MRI, ultrasound, or a combination to find the cause of the obstruction. However, the "powers that be" may not approve these tests without the results of other tests, such as a CBC and a Liver Panel.

Camp Rothenberg Infirmary
Complete Blood Cell Count (CBC)

PARAMETER	PATIENT RESULT	NORMAL RANGE
WBC X 10^3	9.8	5.0-10.0
%Band	1	1-3
%Seg	60	50-62
%Eosin	1	1-4
%Baso	0	0-1
%Mono	0	0-5
%Lymph	38	25-45
RBC X 10^6	nl	4.5-5.5
Hb g/dl	nl	M 14.0-17.4 F 12.0-16.0
Hct (%)	nl	M 36-48 F 42-52
MCV (fl)	nl	84-96
MCH pg	nl	28-34
MCHC g/dl	nl	32-36
Plts X 10^3	nl	140-400

QUESTIONS

1. What are the lab findings?
2. How, if at all, do these help you further differentiate the cause of her jaundice?
3. What general condition (in terms of mechanism) is likely present?
4. What would you expect to see on the Liver Panel?

ANSWERS

1.   What are the lab findings?

The CBC is completely normal.

2.   How, if at all, do these help you further differentiate the cause of her jaundice?

The results of the CBC contribute nothing further, other than providing reassurance, to the diagnostic work-up of this woman.

3.   What general condition (in terms of mechanism) is likely present?

My mind remains unchanged – the patient has obstructive jaundice, presumably complete, until proven otherwise. Considering the fact that she had a laparoscopic cholecystectomy 8 months ago, a retained common duct stone is certainly a possibility. However, the possibility of a tumor (especially of the pancreas) or other obstructing lesion must still be excluded.

4.   What would you expect to see on the Liver Panel?

Since the patient is clinically jaundiced, the total bilirubin should be up. Most of it should be conjugated, since bilirubinuria is present. Since alkaline phosphatase is excreted by the liver, obstruction should raise this measurement as well. Finally, ALT/AST (SGPT/SGOT) are not over twice normal in the face of pure obstruction. Let's see what the results show.

Camp Rothenberg Infirmary
Liver Panel

Parameter	Patient result	Normal value (adults)
Bilirubin, total	5.0	0.2-1.0 mg/dl
Bilirubin, direct (conjugated)	4.5	0.0-0.2 mg/dl
Bilirubin, indirect (unconjugated)	0.5	0.2-0.8 mg/dl
Alanine transaminase (ALT, SGPT [serum glutamic-pyruvic transaminase])	60	7-56 U/L
Alkaline phosphatase (ALP)	300	17-142 IU/L
Aspartate transaminase (AST; serum glutamic-oxaloacetic transaminase [SGOT])	45	5-40 U/L

QUESTIONS

1. What are the lab findings?
2. Are they compatible with the presumptive diagnoses discussed above?
3. What other tests might you consider obtaining?

ANSWERS

1. **What are the lab findings?**

   The total bilirubin is elevated, as would be expected in the face of clinical jaundice. The majority of the elevation consists of conjugated bilirubin. Alkaline phosphatase is increased significantly, while ALT/AST (SGPT/SGOT) are only slightly elevated.

2. **Are they compatible with the presumptive diagnoses discussed above?**

   Yes – elevations in the ALT/AST (SGPT/SGOT) are minimal and certainly compatible with obstruction. These enzymes may rise slightly, but are nearly always less than twice normal when obstruction is present. As expected, however, alkaline phosphatase is moderately elevated.

3. **What other tests might you consider obtaining?**

   This patient needs either a CT, MRI, or an ultrasound as soon as possible to determine the exact cause of her problem. If a retained common duct stone is noted, repeated operation may be required.

CASE 11

66 year old male complains of epigastric pain off and on for a month. He appears somewhat emaciated and you wonder if he is slightly icteric.

Camp Rothenberg Infirmary
Urinalysis (UA)

PARAMETER	PATIENT RESULT	NORMAL RANGE
Color	Orange	Pale yellow to amber
Appearance	Clear	Clear to slightly hazy
Specific gravity	1.015	1.015-1.025
pH	5.0	4.5-8.0
Glucose	-	Negative
Ketones	-	Negative
Blood	-	Negative
Protein	-	Negative
Bilirubin	+++	Negative
Urobilinogen	-	Negative-trace
Nitrate for bacteria	-	Negative
Leucocyte esterase	-	Negative
Casts	-	Negative
RBC	-	Rare or negative
WBC	-	Negative or rare
Crystals	-	Negative
Epithelial cells	-	Few
Bacteria	-	None

QUESTIONS

1.   What are the lab findings?
2.   Mechanistically, what do these suggest regarding the hepatobiliary system?
3.   What additional lab tests do you want to obtain?
4.   How does the above patient differ from the patient presented in Case 10?

ANSWERS

1.   What are the lab findings?

The UA demonstrates two abnormalities – abnormal color (orange) and 3+ bilirubinuria. Note that no urobilinogen is present in the urine.

2.   Mechanistically, what do these suggest regarding the hepatobiliary system?

Remember, when you see a "yellow fellow," give 'em a cup and do a "dip UA." The presence of bilirubin in the urine is always abnormal – to appear in the urine, bilirubin must first be conjugated (water-soluble). In addition, bilirubin in the urine must never have gotten to the bowel in the first place – if it did, it would be converted into urobilinogen and be passed in either the feces (as "brown dye #2") or in the urine (as urinary urobilinogen). As we've said earlier, bilirubinuria indicates some type of liver or biliary drainage system problem – hepatobiliary disease. There are only two generic mechanisms whereby bilirubin can 1) be conjugated and 2) *not* pass into the bowel (see Case 8) – failure of hepatic secretion (e.g., hepatitis, toxin) or obstruction (complete or partial).

In this case, our patient has intermittent epigastric pain, scleral icterus, large amounts of bilirubin in the urine, and no detectable urobilinogen. The combination is worrisome and, until proven otherwise, indicates complete obstruction somewhere in the hepatobiliary drainage system.

3.   What additional lab tests do you want to obtain?

My personal opinion is that there are no lab tests that will change my mind at this point – the patient needs a CT scan, MRI, ultrasound, or a combination to find the cause of the obstruction. However, the "powers that be" may not approve these tests without the results of other tests, such as a CBC and a Liver Panel. I would expect the CBC and Liver Panel results to be similar to those found in Case 10.

4.   How does the above patient differ from the patient presented in Case 10?

The major differences between the patient in Case 10 and in this case are the sex, age, and clinical circumstances. The laboratory profiles are nearly identical. Though other causes must still be diligently sought, the lady in Case 10 has a possible "obvious" explanation for her problem – a post-cholescystectomy complication, such as a retained common duct stone. The gentleman in the current case above has no such history. In addition, he appears "somewhat emaciated." This clinical picture, combined with a laboratory picture favoring complete hepatobiliary obstruction, suggests pancreatic cancer until proven otherwise. The work-up for this man should proceed expeditiously in the same manner as that for the lady in Case 10.

CASE 12

17 year old white female presents with nausea, vomiting, weakness for two days. Mild mid-abdominal pain; no vaginal discharge; serum pregnancy test is negative.

Camp Rothenberg Infirmary
Chemistry Panel

Test	Patient result	Normal value (adult)
Sodium (Na$^+$)	147	135-145 mEq/L
Potassium (K$^+$)	4.0	3.5-5.3 mEq/L
Chloride (Cl$^-$)	108	98-106 mEq/L
Bicarbonate (HCO$_3^-$)	12	23-30 mmol/L
Calcium (Ca^{2+})	9.0	8.6-10.0 mg/dl
Magnesium (Mg^{2+})	1.7	1.3-2.1 mEq/L
Blood sugar (BS)	750	65-110 mg/dl
Blood urea nitrogen (BUN)	35	7-18 mg/dl
Creatinine (Cr)	1.8	0.6-1.3 mg/dl
Uric acid	7.0	Men: 3.5-7.2 mg/dl; women: 2.6-6.0 mg/dl

QUESTIONS

1. What are the lab findings?
2. Which, if any, of the above tests suggest that the patient is dehydrated?
3. What other laboratory tests could be obtained that would support the diagnosis of dehydration?
4. What is the patient's pH?
5. What are possible causes for the patient's acid-base disturbance?
6. What lab test(s) could be used to narrow down the diagnostic possibilities?

ANSWERS

1. What are the lab findings?

There are elevations of the following parameters: sodium, chloride, blood sugar, BUN, and Cr. The bicarbonate is low.

2. Which, if any, of the above tests suggest that the patient is dehydrated?

Of all the electrolytes, serum sodium concentration is the most sensitive to the patient's hydration status. The mild elevation noted here is compatible with dehydration, but other causes cannot be excluded. Elevated BUN and Cr, especially with the BUN/Cr ratio greater than 10, suggests pre-renal azotemia, often due to dehydration. Of course, the clinical picture (nausea and vomiting with weakness) is compatible with the laboratory findings.

3. What other laboratory tests could be obtained that would support the diagnosis of dehydration?

When dehydration occurs, regardless of the cause, hemoconcentration is present. This is reflected not only in the chemistry panel (sodium, BUN, Cr) but in the CBC and the urinalysis. In the CBC, the H/H are often mildly increased; less often, the WBC and platelet counts are similarly affected. On the UA, the urine specific gravity is increased with dehydration. Sometimes the dipstick will show ketones in the urine; however, measurement of serum ketones in patients with dehydration alone (i.e., no other cause) is usually negative.

4. What is the patient's pH?

Trick question (sort of!) – there is no way on the chemistry panel to determine the patient's pH – nor is there usually a need. Note that the bicarbonate level is low. This *defines* the presence of a metabolic acidosis. The process is present whether the net serum pH is high, low, or normal. Remember that bicarbonate represents "metabolic base" and is regulated primarily through the kidneys. Thus, changes in pH in response to changes in the bicarbonate level take hours to days. Also, respiratory compensation for metabolic problems (acidosis or alkalosis) occurs fairly quickly – this is likely to alter the pH, if measured, such that it doesn't directly reflect the severity of the metabolic acidosis directly. Most of the clinical implications in treatment of patients with metabolic acidoses (e.g., serum potassium levels) apply when a metabolic acidosis is determined to be present based on the bicarbonate level, regardless of the pH.

5.   What are possible causes for the patient's acid-base disturbance?

A common way to classify metabolic acidosis is to determine whether an anion gap is present. This calculation reflects concentrations of unmeasured anions that are present in the extracellular fluid (ECF) (e.g., phosphates, sulfates, ketone bodies, lactate, and proteins) to maintain electrical neutrality. Their levels increase in certain types of metabolic acidoses. The formula is as follows:

$$\text{Anion Gap (AG)} = (Na^+ + K^+) - (Cl^- + HCO_3^-) \text{ [normal} = < 16 \text{ mEq/L]}$$

The normal value is 16. In the current case, we calculate the anion gap using the patient's electrolyte values as follows:

$$AG = (147 + 4) - (108 + 12) = 151 - 120 = 31$$

So, the patient has a widened anion gap – this indicates that her body is producing excess metabolic acids. The acronym for various causes of a widened anion gap metabolic acidosis is "SLUMPED:"

S --	Salicylate intoxication
L --	Lactic acidosis
U --	Uremia (renal failure), underfed (fasting, starvation)
M --	Methanol ingestion
P --	Paraldehyde OD (rare)
E --	Ethanol (alcoholic ketoacidosis), ethylene glycol ingestion
D --	Diabetic ketoacidosis

So, any of the above conditions *could* be present. The question becomes: "which is the most likely?"

6.   What lab test(s) could be used to narrow down the diagnostic possibilities?

In light of the clinical history and the elevated blood sugar, I'd bet on diabetic ketoacidosis (DKA) as being the most likely possibility. The easiest way to confirm this, laboratory-wise, is to obtain a serum ketone level. Urine ketones are very nonspecific – they go up with very mild dehydration from any reason, in low-carbohydrate diets, and in both alcoholic and diabetic ketoacidosis. An elevated serum ketone level, however, in the face of elevated blood sugar and clinical findings, is essentially diagnostic of DKA.

CASE 13

25 year-old male complains of severe leg cramps, weakness, and nausea after working on a hot roof for 4 hours. The outside temperature is 100 degrees, the humidity 98%. The patient has been drinking diet soda for fluid replenishment.

Camp Rothenberg Infirmary
Chemistry Panel

Test	Patient result	Normal value (adult)
Sodium (Na$^+$)	160	135-145 mEq/L
Potassium (K$^+$)	5.5	3.5-5.3 mEq/L
Chloride (Cl$^-$)	115	98-106 mEq/L
Bicarbonate (HCO$_3^-$)	22	23-30 mmol/L
Blood sugar (BS)	170	65-110 mg/dl
Blood urea nitrogen (BUN)	65	7-18 mg/dl
Creatinine (Cr)	2.5	0.6-1.3 mg/dl

QUESTIONS

1. What are the lab findings?
2. Which, if any, of the above tests suggest that the patient is dehydrated?
3. What other laboratory tests could be obtained that would support the diagnosis of dehydration?
4. What is the most likely cause of the patient's symptoms and the above laboratory picture?
5. How do you explain the bicarbonate level?

ANSWERS

1. **What are the lab findings?**

   All parameters, except for the bicarbonate level, are significantly elevated.

2. **Which, if any, of the above tests suggest that the patient is dehydrated?**

   Of all the electrolytes, serum sodium concentration is the most sensitive to the patient's hydration status. The large elevation here is highly suggestive of dehydration, regardless of the cause. Elevated BUN and Cr, especially with the BUN/Cr ratio greater than 10, also suggests dehydration. In fact, all of the parameters in this chemistry panel, except for the bicarbonate, are elevated – dehydration is a common cause of generalized elevations in multiple tests (hemoconcentration). Remember that the most common causes of laboratory abnormalities are fluids and drugs!

3. **What other laboratory tests could be obtained that would support the diagnosis of dehydration?**

   When dehydration occurs, regardless of the cause, hemoconcentration is present. This is reflected not only in the chemistry panel but also in the CBC and the urinalysis. In the CBC, the H/H are often mildly increased; less often, the WBC and platelet counts are similarly affected. On the UA, the urine specific gravity is increased with dehydration. Sometimes the dipstick will show ketones in the urine; however, measurement of serum ketones in patients with dehydration alone (i.e., no other cause) is usually negative.

4. **What is the most likely cause of the patient's symptoms and the above laboratory picture?**

   Clinically, the patient has heat cramps and moderate heat exhaustion. Both are caused by excessive sweating in an unacclimatized patient, usually with inappropriate/inadequate fluid replacement. Fluid and salt are lost together in the sweat; replacement with diet soda doesn't contain the same electrolyte mix as sweat. In this case, inadequate free water was taken in by the patient, allowing the sodium concentration (as well as the concentration of most of the other electrolytes) to rise considerably. Part of the elevated BUN/Cr reflects a hemoconcentration effect, though most of the change is directly due to renal hypoperfusion from hypovolemia due to excess fluid loss (and inadequate replacement).

5.   **How do you explain the bicarbonate level?**

Tissue hypoperfusion as a result of hemoconcentration probably resulted in a small amount of anaerobic metabolism in some cells. In addition, the massive muscle spasm due to the electrolyte abnormality also led to the production of lactic acid in the muscles. This combination could easily produce a mild metabolic acidosis.

CASE 14

74 year old white male, 5 days following radical head/neck surgery for carcinoma. Has taken nothing via NG tube or mouth; IV fluids only since surgery, mostly consisting of D5W-1/4NaCl. On rounds, you notice that the patient is markedly less responsive than when you last saw him.

Camp Rothenberg Infirmary
Chemistry Panel

Test	Patient result	Normal value (adult)
Sodium (Na$^+$)	105	135-145 mEq/L
Potassium (K$^+$)	3.0	3.5-5.3 mEq/L
Chloride (Cl$^-$)	78	98-106 mEq/L
Bicarbonate (HCO$_3^-$)	35	23-30 mmol/L
Blood sugar (BS)	60	65-110 mg/dl
Blood urea nitrogen (BUN)	5.0	7-18 mg/dl
Creatinine (Cr)	0.8	0.6-1.3 mg/dl

QUESTIONS

1. What are the lab findings?
2. What is the most likely cause of the patient's symptoms and the above laboratory picture?
3. How would you explain the BUN and Cr levels?
4. How would you explain the bicarbonate level?
5. Over what period of time would you correct the patient's electrolyte abnormalities?

ANSWERS

1. **What are the lab findings?**

    All measured parameters on the Chemistry Panel, except for the bicarbonate, are significantly lower than normal. The bicarbonate is moderately elevated.

2. **What is the most likely cause of the patient's symptoms and the above laboratory picture?**

    Though the syndrome of inappropriate ADH secretion (SIADH) due to the patient's underlying cancer cannot be excluded, there seems to be a far more obvious cause of these abnormalities – poor nutrition, combined with inappropriate IV fluid administration. Recall that there is an obligate 40 meq per day urinary potassium loss – since the patient received nothing by mouth and the was no potassium in his IV fluids, I'm not a bit surprised that hypokalemia is present. Add to this the dilutional component of D5W-1/4NaCl – essentially free water. This solution is significantly hypotonic to normal serum and has diluted nearly all of the major electrolytes. This situation is likely iatrogenic and probably was avoidable.

3. **How would you explain the BUN and Cr levels?**

    The Cr is unremarkable – the low BUN could be due to severe liver disease and failure to appropriately metabolize protein, but there is no other evidence for this. The most likely cause of the low BUN is poor intake – essentially, this patient has been starving for five days. Low dietary intake of protein is a well-documented cause of low BUN.

4. **How would you explain the bicarbonate level?**

    Though there are several potential explanations for the patient's metabolic alkalosis, the most likely is NG suction. This removes gastric acid. Especially in the face of poor nutrition, the body is unable to re-establish normal acid-base balance.

5. **Over what period of time would you correct the patient's electrolyte abnormalities?**

    It's taken several days for the observed metabolic abnormalities to become established. The low serum sodium level has likely resulted in a significant change in serum osmolality. Since this occurred relatively slowly, the cerebrospinal fluid (CSF) osmolality has probably equilibrated with that of the serum. If we rapidly change the serum sodium level, there will be a marked osmotic difference between serum and the CSF, precipitating seizures, and even death. So, the general rule is to correct hyponatremia over the time period that you think it took to develop. If it occurred acutely, treatment can proceed rapidly. But, if the hyponatremia took more than 48 hours to occur, take your time!

CASE 15

25 year old male, known diabetic, presents with nausea, vomiting, tachypnea.

Camp Rothenberg Infirmary
"Incomplete" Blood Cell Count (CBC)

PARAMETER	RESULT	NORMAL
WBC X 10³	10.7	5.0-10.0
%Band	4	1-3
%Seg	65	50-62
%Eosin	1	1-4
%Baso	1	0-1
%Mono	1	0-5
%Lymph	28	25-45
Hb g/dl	18	12-17
Hct (%)	54	36-52
MCV (fl)	nl	84-96
MCH pg	nl	28-34
MCHC g/dl	nl	32-36
Plts X 10³	450	140-400

QUESTIONS

1.   What are the lab findings?
2.   What are possible explanations for these findings?
3.   If the above assumption (the most likely explanation) is correct, what would you expect to see on the UA?

ANSWERS

1.   **What are the lab findings?**

The CBC shows a slight elevation in the total WBC count and percentages of segs (neutrophils). H/H and the platelet count are all mildly elevated.

2.   **What are possible explanations for these findings?**

Though we could hypothesize various tumors secreting bone marrow stimulating substances, the most likely explanation for these findings is far simpler. Whenever virtually everything in a set of lab work is either uniformly increased or decreased, think fluids. Dehydration with hemoconcentration could easily explain the entire picture. Another possible explanation is chronic hypoxia, including cigarette smoking. This leads to the production of erythropoietin (by the kidneys), thrombopoietin (by the liver), and leukopoietin (by the liver). A final possibility is polycythemia vera – essentially, a neoplasm of the bone marrow with increased production of all three cell lines – red cells, white cells, and platelets.

3.   **If the above assumption (the most likely explanation) is correct, what would you expect to see on the UA?**

If dehydration (hypovolemia) was the cause of the above CBC, we'd expect the specific gravity in the urine to be elevated. In addition, there may be ketones present.

Camp Rothenberg Infirmary
Urinalysis (UA)

TEST	PATIENT	NORMAL
Color	yellow	Pale yellow to amber
Appearance	sl cloudy	Clear to slightly hazy
Specific gravity	1.027	1.015-1.025
pH	5.0	4.5-8.0
Glucose	++	Negative
Ketones	+	Negative
Blood	-	Negative
Protein	+	Negative
Bilirubin	-	Negative
Urobilinogen	-	Negative-trace
Nitrate for bacteria	-	Negative
Leucocyte esterase	-	Negative
Casts	-	Negative
RBC	-	Rare or negative
WBC	-	Negative or rare
Crystals	-	Negative
Epithelial cells	few	Few
Bacteria	-	None

QUESTIONS

1.   What are the lab findings?
2.   Are they compatible with dehydration?
3.   How would you explain the glucose level?
4.   How would you explain the protein level?

ANSWERS

1. **What are the lab findings?**

The specific gravity is increased. On the dipstick, glucose is 2+, ketones 1+, and protein 1+. Other than a few epithelial cells seen on the microscopic exam, the remainder of the UA is unremarkable.

2. **Are they compatible with dehydration?**

Yes – the findings of increased specific gravity and small amounts of ketones are commonly caused by dehydration. Another possible reason for ketones in the urine is diabetic ketoacidosis (DKA). However, this must be verified by measurement of serum ketones to diagnose DKA.

3. **How would you explain the glucose level?**

Mild glucosuria may occur in anyone, especially during periods of stress. Recall that there is essentially little to no correlation between a person's urine sugar level and his or her blood sugar. This is true in everyone – not just in diabetics. Yes, it's possible that this patient's urine glucose is elevated due to an elevated blood sugar, but it's just as likely that there isn't a direct relationship.

4. **How would you explain the protein level?**

Dehydration, per se, should not cause the glucose level in the urine to rise. The slight elevation in the urinary protein, however, *is* likely a reflection of dehydration. If there is a small amount of protein in the patient's urine normally (say, from early diabetic nephropathy), dehydration will concentrate the urine and make the concentration of protein look even larger. With low levels of proteinuria, especially in a diabetic, a 24-hour urine collection for total protein determination is necessary before reaching any major conclusions regarding proteinuria.

Camp Rothenberg Infirmary
Chemistry Panel

Test	Patient	Normal
Sodium (Na$^+$)	145	135-145 mEq/L
Potassium (K$^+$)	3.4	3.5-5.3 mEq/L
Chloride (Cl$^-$)	105	98-106 mEq/L
Bicarbonate (HCO$_3^-$)	13	23-30 mmol/L
Blood sugar (BS)	400	65-110 mg/dl
Blood urea nitrogen (BUN)	22	7-18 mg/dl
Creatinine (Cr)	1.6	0.6-1.3 mg/dl

QUESTIONS

1.   What are the lab findings?
2.   Which, if any, of the above tests suggest that the patient is dehydrated?
3.   What other laboratory tests could be obtained that would support the diagnosis of dehydration?
4.   What are possible causes for the patient's acid-base disturbance?
5.   What lab test(s) could be used to narrow down the diagnostic possibilities?
6.   Discuss the significance of the potassium level in regards to the above diagnostic possibilities (hint – what does the low bicarbonate level imply?).
7.   Are arterial blood gases necessary to properly manage this patient?

QUESTIONS

1. **What are the lab findings?**

The blood sugar, BUN, and Cr are elevated. The potassium and bicarbonate are low.

2. **Which, if any, of the above tests suggest that the patient is dehydrated?**

Elevation of the BUN with slight increase in the Cr, and a BUN/Cr ratio of > 10 suggests dehydration.

3. **What other laboratory tests could be obtained that would support the diagnosis of dehydration?**

The specific gravity would be increased on the UA and small amounts of ketones may be present. Depending upon the degree of dehydration, the CBC may show increases in all three cell line measurements: H/H, WBC count, and platelet count.

4. **What are possible causes for the patient's acid-base disturbance?**

A common way to classify metabolic acidosis is to determine whether an anion gap is present. This calculation reflects concentrations of unmeasured anions that are present in the ECF (e.g., phosphates, sulfates, ketone bodies, lactate, and proteins) to maintain electrical neutrality. Their levels increase in certain types of metabolic acidoses. The formula is as follows:

$$\textbf{Anion Gap (AG)} = (Na^+ + K^+) - (Cl^- + HCO_3^-) \textbf{ [normal} = < 16 \textbf{ mEq/L]}$$

The normal value is 16. In the current case, we calculate the anion gap using the patient's electrolyte values as follows:

$$AG = (145 + 3.4) - (105 + 13) = 148.4 - 118 = 30.4$$

So, the patient has a widened anion gap – this indicates that his body is producing excess metabolic acids. The acronym for various causes of a widened anion gap metabolic acidosis is "SLUMPED:"

S --	Salicylate intoxication
L --	Lactic acidosis
U --	Uremia (renal failure), underfed (fasting, starvation)
M --	Methanol ingestion
P --	Paraldehyde OD (rare)
E --	Ethanol (alcoholic ketoacidosis), ethylene glycol ingestion
D --	Diabetic ketoacidosis

So, any of the above conditions *could* be present. The question becomes: "which is the most likely?"

5.   What lab test(s) could be used to narrow down the diagnostic possibilities?

In light of the clinical history and the elevated blood sugar, I'd bet on diabetic ketoacidosis (DKA) as being the most likely possibility. The easiest way to confirm this, laboratory-wise, is to obtain a serum ketone level. Urine ketones are very nonspecific – they go up with very mild dehydration from any reason, in low-carbohydrate diets, and in both alcoholic and diabetic ketoacidosis. An elevated serum ketone level, however, in the face of elevated blood sugar and clinical findings, is essentially diagnostic of DKA.

6.   Discuss the significance of the potassium level in regards to the above diagnostic possibilities (hint – what does the low bicarbonate level imply?).

The low bicarbonate level means that the patient has a metabolic acidosis. And, metabolic acidosis, regardless of the reason and independent of the pH, causes an increase in the serum potassium level (see text). Treatment of the acidosis has the exact opposite effect. This patient's potassium is 3.4 mEq/L prior to treatment – so the "patient safe" assumption is that when we treat the patient, the level will fall even further. It's probably a good idea to give this patient some potassium (add it to the IV fluids and/or IV bolus) *prior* to starting insulin therapy. Remember, insulin shifts potassium into the cells – it's one of the routine treatments for hyperkalemia.

7.   Are arterial blood gases (ABGs) necessary to properly manage this patient?

Opinions on this topic vary widely. Many argue that following the measured bicarbonate level on the Chemistry Panel is sufficient. Others suggest that ABGs be obtained to determine whether or not to administer bicarbonate – despite much data showing that overzealous administration of sodium bicarbonate can be worse than none at all. My personal opinion is to avoid IV sodium bicarbonate in most cases. Localized alkalosis causes the oxyhemoglobin dissociation curve to shift to the left. This results in two undesirable events:

- Increased affinity of hemoglobin for oxygen (hemoglobin "holds on" to oxygen tighter than usual)
- Decreased tissue oxygen delivery (hemoglobin won't "let go" of the oxygen and give it to the tissues as easily)

Having spoken my peace, let's assume that ABGs *were* obtained and see how to use them.

Camp Rothenberg Infirmary
Arterial Blood Gases

Parameter	Patient	Normal
pH	7.20	7.35-7.45
pCO_2	25	35-45 mmHg (torr)
pO_2	85	> 80 mmHg (torr)

QUESTIONS

1. Is the pO_2 low?
2. Which way did the pH go, up or down?
3. Did the pCO_2 move in the *opposite* direction of the pO_2?
4. What is the primary underlying acid-base disorder based on the above three-question approach?
5. Is there evidence for any type of compensatory process?

ANSWERS

1.   Is the pO_2 low?

No, oxygenation is adequate – so we move on, and look at the pH.

2.   Which way did the pH go, up or down?

It went down – this means that the patient is acidotic (implies that the primary process is an acidosis)

3.   Did the pCO_2 move in the *opposite* direction of the pH?

No – since the pCO_2 did not move in the *opposite* direction of the pH, the primary underlying problem is metabolic (see text, Arterial Blood Gases, Chapter 7).

4.   What is the primary underlying acid-base disorder based on the above three-question approach?

The primary problem is a metabolic acidosis with normal room air oxygenation.

5.   Is there evidence for any type of compensatory process?

Yes – the pCO_2 is lower than normal. When a metabolic acidosis occurs, such as is the case here, the body soon responds by hypo- or hyperventilating to compensate, at least partially. Complete compensation does not occur in the acute setting. Remember, pCO_2 is "respiratory acid" and when it changes, the pH changes rapidly – in the opposite direction. Also, recall the "happy marriage," in that for every 10 mm Hg change in the pCO_2, the pH will instantly change 0.1 units in the *opposite direction*.

If we assume 40 mm Hg to be a normal pCO_2 level, then the above patient has compensated by "blowing off" 15 mm Hg of pCO_2 (respiratory acid). Using the 10:0.1 relationship, we conclude that a 15 point *decrease* in the pCO_2 leads to a 0.15 *increase* in the pH. So, if the patient's pH is now 7.20 with compensation, it was roughly 0.15 less, or, 7.05 prior to compensation.

CASE 16

65 year old male, known diabetic, presents with epigastric pain and weakness.

Camp Rothenberg Infirmary
Complete Blood Cell Count (CBC)

PARAMETER	PATIENT	NORMAL
WBC X 10^3	6.0	5.0-10.0
%Band	1	1-3
%Seg	50	50-62
%Eosin	1	1-4
%Baso	1	0-1
%Mono	1	0-5
%Lymph	46	25-45
RBC X 10^6	3.2	4.5-5.5
Hb g/dl	10.5	M 14.0-17.4 F 12.0-16.0
Hct (%)	31.2	M 36-48 F 42-52
MCV (fl)	nl	84-96
MCH pg	nl	28-34
MCHC g/dl	nl	32-36
Plts X 10^3	120	140-400

QUESTIONS

1. What are the lab findings?
2. Regarding the RBC count, what general condition is present?
3. Describe how you would further classify the above condition.
4. What are possible causes of this condition in the above patient?
5. How would you explain the platelet count?

220

ANSWERS

1. What are the lab findings?

STOP!! Consider the clinical history – a 65-year old male diabetic with epigastric discomfort and weakness. As far as I'm concerned, this man has acute myocardial ischemia until proven otherwise – don't you agree? Any work-up done should first center around acute MI and acute coronary syndromes. Having done this – we'll assume whatever work-up necessary was negative – we can proceed.

The WBC and associated parameters are WNL. The RBC, H/H, and platelet count are low, while the MCV is normal.

2. Regarding the RBC count, what general condition is present?

The above findings suggest anemia (decreased numbers of RBCs). We can further classify the type of anemia present, as discussed in the next question.

3. Describe how you would further classify the above condition.

To classify anemias, we determine whether the cells are "ugly" or not – in other words, are they normal sized, too big, or too small? The easiest way to do this is to look at the MCV, a direct reflection of cell size. In this case, the MCV is normal, so the red cells are normal in size. This is termed a normocytic anemia. Normal red cell size suggests that the "intrinsic machinery" of the cell is intact. However, the bone marrow simply isn't making enough of these *normal cells* to keep up with the demand – and the patient becomes anemic.

4. What are possible causes of this condition in the above patient?

The most common causes of normocytic anemia are chronic disease or acute bleeding. The long-standing history of diabetes certainly qualifies as a chronic disease, and could explain the anemia. There is no evidence of massive bleeding, external or internal. However, it's still possible that the patient could have low-grade internal bleeding, accounting for the anemia. Bleeding does not, however, explain the somewhat decreased platelet count.

5. How would you explain the platelet count?

Bleeding, by itself, does not lead to a significant decrease in the platelet count. Can you think of a *single* cause that could result in epigastric pain, weakness, anemia, and a mildly decreased platelet On the next page are the results of the patient's UA and Liver Profile, both of which were normal. In addition, the patient's PT, INR, and PTT were all normal.

Camp Rothenberg Infirmary
Urinalysis (UA)

PARAMETER	PATIENT	NORMAL
Color	dk yellow	Pale yellow to amber
Appearance	slightly hazy	Clear to slightly hazy
Specific gravity	1.023	1.015-1.025
pH	4.7	4.5-8.0
Glucose	-	Negative
Ketones	-	Negative
Blood	-	Negative
Protein	-	Negative
Bilirubin	-	Negative
Urobilinogen	tr	Negative-trace
Nitrate for bacteria	-	Negative
Leucocyte esterase	-	Negative
Casts	-	Negative
RBC	-	Rare or negative
WBC	-	Negative or rare
Crystals	-	Negative
Epithelial cells	-	Few
Bacteria	-	None

Camp Rothenberg Infirmary
Liver Panel

Parameter	Patient result	Normal value (adults)
Bilirubin, total	1.0	0.2-1.0 mg/dl
ALT (SGPT)	45	7-56 U/L
Alkaline phosphatase (ALP)	100	17-142 IU/L
AST (SGOT)	35	5-40 U/L
Lactic acid dehydrogenase (LDH)	340	313-618 U/L

222

Camp Rothenberg Infirmary
Chemistry Panel

Sodium (Na$^+$)	143	135-145 mEq/L
Potassium (K$^+$)	3.7	3.5-5.3 mEq/L
Chloride (Cl$^-$)	105	98-106 mEq/L
Bicarbonate (HCO$_3^-$)	28	23-30 mmol/L
Blood sugar (BS)	140	65-110 mg/dl
Blood urea nitrogen (BUN)	45	7-18 mg/dl
Creatinine (Cr)	1.7	0.6-1.3 mg/dl

QUESTIONS

1. What are the lab findings?
2. Based on the BUN and Cr, could the patient be dehydrated?
3. Do any of the patient's other lab tests support the diagnosis of dehydration?
4. Is there another explanation for the BUN and Cr levels?
5. Can you think of a *single* cause that could result in epigastric pain, weakness, anemia, and a mildly decreased platelet count?

ANSWERS

1.   What are the lab findings?

The Chemistry Panel is normal except for elevations of the blood sugar, BUN, and Cr.

2.   Based on the BUN and Cr, could the patient be dehydrated?

The BUN is elevated out of proportion to the Cr; the BUN/Cr ratio is > 10. These findings are compatible with dehydration. However, no clinical features are noted that suggest dehydration. Let's see if the diagnosis is corroborated by other lab tests.

3.   Do any of the patient's other lab tests support the diagnosis of dehydration?

No – the urine specific gravity is normal and no ketones are present. There is no evidence of hemoconcentration on the CBC.

4.   Is there another explanation for the BUN and Cr levels?

Yes – recall that BUN is derived from protein breakdown. If a patient has poor dietary intake, his or her BUN is usually very low. On the other hand, excessive protein digested in the stomach leads to *increased* levels of BUN. An excellent source of additional protein in the stomach is blood. Upper GI bleeding (UGIB) leads to an elevation of the BUN, without significantly affecting the creatinine. In this case, the creatinine may have been elevated slightly due to mild hypovolemia that is not obvious otherwise, either clinically or on other lab tests.

BUN levels in the face of on-going UGIB are usually in the range of 40 mg/dL or greater, as is the case here. If the bleeding stops, the BUN returns to normal within 24 hours; if bleeding resumes, the BUN increases within 6-8 hours. Placing a nasogastric (NG) tube to determine if there is on-going GI bleeding is only 70% sensitive (i.e., there's a 30% false-negative rate) – many clinicians use BUN levels to follow patients following apparent cessation of UGIB.

5.   Can you think of a *single* cause that could result in epigastric pain, weakness, anemia, and a mildly decreased platelet count?

Non-steroidal anti-inflammatory drugs (NSAIDs), such as ibuprofen, could explain the entire picture. They can cause gastritis and/or peptic ulcer disease – either can result in UGIB. In addition, the NSAIDs often cause mild thrombocytopenia, probably due to bone marrow suppression. They also cause a qualitative platelet defect, prolonging the bleeding time.

As it turns out, the patient was taking large doses (600-800 mg, three to four times daily) of over-the-counter ibuprofen. Upper GI endoscopy showed diffuse gastritis with intermittent oozing of blood from the inflamed stomach mucosa. No ulcers were present. The patient's symptoms and anemia responded well to cessation of ibuprofen, antacids, and H_2-blocker therapy.

By the way, the patient's stool on his initial examination was guiac-positive (heme-positive). I didn't want to tell you this at the beginning of the case because it made finding the diagnosis too easy ☺

CASE 17

13 year old girl presents with hyperactivity, "nervous behavior," and hyperventilation.

Camp Rothenberg Infirmary
Chemistry Panel

Test	Patient result	Normal value (adult)
Sodium (Na^+)	140	135-145 mEq/L
Potassium (K^+)	4.1	3.5-5.3 mEq/L
Chloride (Cl^-)	99	98-106 mEq/L
Bicarbonate (HCO_3^-)	12	23-30 mmol/L
Blood sugar (BS)	100	65-110 mg/dl
Blood urea nitrogen (BUN)	8	7-18 mg/dl
Creatinine (Cr)	0.7	0.6-1.3 mg/dl

QUESTIONS

1. What are the lab findings?
2. What is the significance of the bicarbonate level?
3. What are possible causes for the patient's acid-base disturbance?

ANSWERS

1. **What are the lab findings?**

The Chemistry Panel is WNL except for a significantly decreased bicarbonate level.

2. **What is the significance of the bicarbonate level?**

It is decreased, indicating that the patient has a metabolic acidosis. Remember, that this process is identified by the presence of a *low measured bicarbonate level*, not by the pH on an arterial blood gas (ABG).

3. **What are possible causes for the patient's acid-base disturbance?**

A common way to classify metabolic acidosis is to determine whether an anion gap is present. This calculation reflects concentrations of unmeasured anions that are present in the ECF (e.g., phosphates, sulfates, ketone bodies, lactate, and proteins) to maintain electrical neutrality. Their levels increase in certain types of metabolic acidoses. The formula is as follows:

$$\textbf{Anion Gap (AG)} = (Na^+ + K^+) - (Cl^- + HCO_3^-) \; [\textbf{normal} = < 16 \; \textbf{mEq/L}]$$

The normal value is 16. In the current case, we calculate the anion gap using the patient's electrolyte values as follows:

$$AG = (140 + 4.1) - (99 + 12) = 144.1 - 111 = 33.1$$

So, the patient has a widened anion gap – this indicates that her body is producing excess metabolic acids. The acronym for various causes of a widened anion gap metabolic acidosis is "SLUMPED:"

S --	Salicylate intoxication
L --	Lactic acidosis
U --	Uremia (renal failure), underfed (fasting, starvation)
M --	Methanol ingestion
P --	Paraldehyde OD (rare)
E --	Ethanol (alcoholic ketoacidosis), ethylene glycol ingestion
D --	Diabetic ketoacidosis

So, any of the above conditions *could* be present. The question becomes: "which is the most likely?" Because of a confusing clinical picture, the patient's health care providers felt that an ABG might be helpful. The results are shown on the next page.

227

Camp Rothenberg Infirmary
Arterial Blood Gases

Parameter	Patient	Normal
pH	7.50	7.35-7.45
pCO_2	20	35-45 mmHg (torr)
pO_2	100	> 80 mmHg (torr)

QUESTIONS

1. Is the pO_2 low?
2. Which way did the pH go, up or down?
3. Did the pCO_2 move in the *opposite* direction of the pO_2?
4. What is the primary underlying acid-base disorder based on the above three-question approach?
5. Is there evidence for any type of compensatory or secondary process?
6. What diagnosis do the above ABG results suggest, based on the "SLUMPED" acronym?

ANSWERS

1.   Is the pO_2 low?

No, oxygenation is adequate – so we move on, and look at the pH.

2.   Which way did the pH go, up or down?

It went up – this means that the patient is alkalotic (implies that the primary process is an alkalosis)

3.   Did the pCO_2 move in the *opposite* direction of the pH?

Yes – since the pCO_2 moved in the *opposite* direction of the pH, the primary underlying problem is respiratory (see text, Arterial Blood Gases, Chapter 7).

4.   What is the primary underlying acid-base disorder based on the above three-question approach?

The primary problem is a respiratory alkalosis with normal oxygenation.

5.   Is there evidence for any type of compensatory or secondary process process?

Yes – if we use 7.40 as the normal pH and 40 mm Hg as the normal pCO_2 – a 20 mm Hg decrease in the pCO_2 should result in a .2 unit *increase* in the pH. So, if the patient had a pure respiratory alkalosis, her pH should be 7.60, *not* 7.50. The pH is *lower* than predicted from the pCO_2 level by .1 units. For this to happen, there must be a concomitant metabolic acidosis acting to lower the pH. This is reflected in the lowered bicarbonate value on the Chemistry Panel above. So, the patient has a combination of a respiratory alkalosis (primary disorder) and a metabolic acidosis (secondary disorder).

6.   What diagnosis do the above ABG results suggest, based on the "SLUMPED" acronym?

The most likely possibility is salicylate (aspirin) intoxication. Initially, salicylates stimulate the respiratory system, resulting in hyperventilation. This leads to a decrease in the pCO_2 level, and a respiratory alkalosis. Salicylates then cause uncoupling of oxidative phosphorylation, preventing cells from adequately using oxygen. The result is a conversion of a portion of the body's cells to anaerobic metabolism with lactic acid production. This causes a metabolic acidosis. So, the "textbook" picture of acute salicylate intoxication is an initial respiratory alkalosis (hyperventilation), followed by a concomitant metabolic acidosis with tissue hypoxia. A serum salicylate level (80 mg/dL) confirmed the diagnosis.

CASE 18

42 year old male on dialysis – presents with weakness.

Camp Rothenberg Infirmary
Complete Blood Cell Count (CBC)

TEST	PATIENT	NORMAL
WBC X 10^3	6.0	5.0-10.0
%Band	0	1-3
%Seg	50	50-62
%Eosin	1	1-4
%Baso	1	0-1
%Mono	1	0-5
%Lymph	47	25-45
RBC X 10^6	3.7	4.5-5.5
Hb g/dl	10.5	12-17
Hct (%)	32	36-52
MCV (fl)	nl	84-96
MCH pg	nl	28-34
MCHC g/dl	nl	32-36
Plts X 10^3	135	140-400

QUESTIONS

1. What are the lab findings?
2. What is the significance of the platelet count?
3. Regarding the RBC count, what general condition is present?
4. Describe how you would further classify the above condition.
5. What are possible causes of this condition in the above patient?
6. What other lab tests might you obtain to further evaluate the patient's weakness?

ANSWERS

1. What are the lab findings?

The WBC count and differential are normal. The RBC count (RBC), hemoglobin (Hb) and hematocrit (Hct) are all low; the MCV and the MCH are normal. The platelet count is mildly decreased.

2. What is the significance of the platelet count?

The slightly decreased platelet count, by itself, is of little clinical significance. However, patients with renal failure tend to have platelet dysfunction – their platelets don't aggregate as well as those in normal persons. So, even with a normal platelet count, these individuals can have bleeding problems – usually, these are minor. They can only be detected if we perform a bleeding time or platelet aggregation tests on the patient. The positive upshot of the platelet problem – patients with chronic renal failure (CRF) tend to have a lower incidence of thromboembolic disease (e.g., pulmonary emboli) than other persons with chronic disease. This may be due to the fact that their platelets are less likely to aggregate, reducing the incidence of thrombus formation.

3. Regarding the RBC count, what general condition is present?

The above findings suggest anemia (decreased numbers of RBCs). We can further classify the type of anemia present, as discussed in the next question.

4. Describe how you would further classify the above condition.

To classify anemias, we determine whether the cells are "ugly" or not – in other words, are they normal sized, too big, or too small? The easiest way to do this is to look at the MCV, a direct reflection of cell size. In this case, the MCV is normal, so the red cells are normal in size. This is termed a normocytic anemia. Normal red cell size suggests that the "intrinsic machinery" of the cell is intact. However, the bone marrow simply isn't making enough of these *normal cells* to keep up with the demand – and the patient becomes anemic.

5. What are possible causes of this condition in the above patient?

The most common causes of normocytic anemia are chronic disease or acute bleeding. Based on the patient's history, acute bleeding is unlikely. Chronic renal failure (CRF) may cause normocytic anemia. In the case of CRF, regardless of the cause, the patient's failing kidneys don't produce enough erythropoietin to sustain normal bone marrow activity. As a result, the patient has a chronic low grade anemia. In fact, many clinicians refer to patients with CRF as being members of the "10/30 Club," meaning that their usual *baseline* Hb is around 10, and the Hct around 30.

Remember, there is a difference between *baseline* and *normal*. Patients with CRF are not expected to have normal values of H/H. Rather, when they are relatively stable (at their baseline), they run an H/H of 10/30. So, if you see a CRF patient whose H/H is significantly lower than 10/30 (i.e., 7/21), don't attribute the anemia to CRF alone. This is *way below* the average for renal failure patients and suggests an additional cause, usually bleeding. The anemia, by itself, may account for the patient's weakness.

6. **What other lab tests might you obtain to further evaluate the patient's weakness?**

Tests of interest would include urinalysis (if the patient still makes some urine) and a chemistry panel. The results of these are shown below and discussed further.

Urinalysis (UA)

TEST	PATIENT	NORMAL
Color	yellow	Pale yellow to amber
Appearance	cloudy	Clear to slightly hazy
SG	1.010	1.015-1.025
pH	7.2	4.5-8.0
Glucose	-	Negative
Ketones	-	Negative
Blood	+	Negative
Protein	+++	Negative
Bilirubin	-	Negative
Urobilinogen	-	Negative-trace
Nitrate for bacteria	-	Negative
Leucocyte esterase	-	Negative
Casts	Hyaline, waxy	Negative
RBC	few	Rare or negative
WBC	-	Negative or rare
Crystals	rare amorphous	Negative
Epithelial cells	few-mod	Few
Bacteria	-	None

QUESTIONS

1.   What are the lab findings?
2.   How can you do a UA on a dialysis patient with CRF?
3.   What is the significance of the specific gravity level in this patient?
4.   What is the significance of blood and protein on the dipstick test?
5.   What is the significance of the casts?
6.   How does the above UA fit into our work-up and treatment of this patient?

1. **What are the lab findings?**

The specific gravity is low; dipstick is positive for 1+ blood and 3+ protein; several different types of casts are present.

2. **How can you do a UA on a dialysis patient with CRF?**

A common misconception is that all persons with CRF are anuric – this is simply not so. Many patients make a small amount of urine – some make nearly normal quantities. However, examination of the urine reveals that it is far from normal otherwise.

3. **What is the significance of the specific gravity level in this patient?**

In a normal person, a specific gravity (SG) of 1.010 may indicate fluid overload. This is also possible in the patient with CRF. However, knowing that the patient's renal function is bad enough to require hemodialysis, there is another more likely explanation – isosthenuria – a condition in which the kidneys produce urine with the specific gravity of protein-free blood plasma. Clinically, this appears as constant SG = 1.010 on repeated urinalyses, regardless of the underlying conditions. Isosthenuria indicates that the patient's kidneys are no longer able to concentrate the urine – a major part of normal renal function. This is compatible with CRF, though not present in all patients.

4. **What is the significance of blood and protein on the dipstick test?**

In a previously normal patient, blood and protein (especially 3+) would be highly bothersome, suggesting acute nephrotic syndrome or severe glomerulonephritis. In patients with CRF, this finding, though abnormal, is not terribly surprising.

5. **What is the significance of the casts?**

Multiple casts, especially a mix of hyaline and waxy casts, are compatible with CRF. Waxy casts are often referred to as "renal failure casts." Other than identifying a patient with renal failure, they add little to the evaluation and treatment of the patient.

6. **How does the above UA fit into our work-up and treatment of this patient?**

It's important to understand what the UA of a patient with CRF usually looks like – and the above urine specimen typifies the *baseline* of most patients with CRF who make urine. As abnormal as it would be in a normal individual, the above findings are often *expected* in patients with CRF. Remember – there is a difference between *normal* and *baseline*.

Camp Rothenberg Infirmary
Chemistry Panel

Test	Patient	Normal
Sodium (Na$^+$)	135	135-145 mEq/L
Potassium (K$^+$)	5.6	3.5-5.3 mEq/L
Chloride (Cl$^-$)	104	98-106 mEq/L
Bicarbonate (HCO$_3^-$)	21	23-30 mmol/L
Blood sugar (BS)	109	65-110 mg/dl
BUN	75	7-18 mg/dl
Creatinine (Cr)	8.2	0.6-1.3 mg/dl

QUESTIONS

1. What are the lab findings?
2. What is the significance of the potassium level?
3. What is the significance of the bicarbonate level?
4. What is the significance of the BUN and Cr levels?
5. Do you expect dialysis to normalize the BUN and Cr levels in this patient?
6. What conclusions can be reached regarding the lab studies we've reviewed in this patient and their relationship to his chief complaint of weakness?

ANSWERS

1. **What are the lab findings?**

   The potassium, BUN, and Cr levels are all elevated. The bicarbonate is low.

2. **What is the significance of the potassium level?**

   A potassium level of 5.6 mEq/L is rarely life-threatening. The only reason to directly treat this low level of hyperkalemia would be if there was evidence of cardiac membrane toxicity – dysrhythmias and/or EKG changes (see Potassium [hyperkalemia], Chapter 4). Mild elevations of potassium are common in CRF patients, especially as they approach the time for their next dialysis.

3. **What is the significance of the bicarbonate level?**

   The kidneys normally excrete excess metabolic acids. When CRF develops, this process is hampered. The result is an abnormal accumulation of metabolic acids, leading to a variable degree of metabolic acidosis. Usually, the pH is not significantly altered due to respiratory compensation. However, the presence of the metabolic acidosis may still be detected by the decreased bicarbonate level. The level tends to rise towards normal following dialysis.

4. **What is the significance of the BUN and Cr levels?**

   Elevation of the BUN and Cr suggest renal dysfunction. The degree of elevation seen in this patient, combined with the BUN/Cr ratio < 10, is compatible with CRF. It is wholly possible that these significant elevations, which would be grossly abnormal in a previously normal individual, may simply represent this patient's *baseline* values prior to dialysis.

5. **Do you expect dialysis to normalize the BUN and Cr levels in this patient?**

   Patients with CRF who require dialysis have poor underlying renal function – the best dialysis can be expected to do is to improve the situation, including patient symptoms. It is unusual for a dialysis session to completely normalize a patient's BUN and creatinine. The only way to do this is by renal transplantation.

6. **What conclusions can be reached regarding the lab studies we've reviewed in this patient and their relationship to his chief complaint of weakness?**

   The entire laboratory picture presented in this case represents typical *baseline* findings in an average CRF patient prior to the next dialysis session. As compared to persons with normal renal function, these studies are grossly abnormal. However, they are *expected findings*, in most CRF patients, especially prior to dialysis.

CASE 19

24 year old female complains of nausea, vomiting, diarrhea for three days. Her serum pregnancy test is negative.

Camp Rothenberg Infirmary
Complete Blood Cell Count (CBC)

TEST	PATIENT	NORMAL
WBC X 10^3	11.3	5.0-10.0
%Band	1	1-3
%Seg	45	50-62
%Eosin	0	1-4
%Baso	0	0-1
%Mono	1	0-5
%Lymph	53	25-45
RBC X 10^6	4.7	4.5-5.5
Hb g/dl	15	12-17
Hct (%)	45	36-52
MCV (fl)	nl	84-96
MCH pg	nl	28-34
MCHC g/dl	nl	32-36
Plts X 10^3	250	140-400

QUESTIONS

1. What are the lab findings?
2. What is the significance of the above findings in regards to the patient's symptoms?
3. Does the CBC suggest that the patient might be dehydrated?
4. If the patient is dehydrated, what other lab tests might help support the diagnosis? What would you expect to find?

ANSWERS

1. **What are the lab findings?**

   NOTE: The most important lab test in women of childbearing age, especially with nausea, vomiting, and/or abdominal pain is the serum pregnancy test. Missed ectopic pregnancy can be fatal.

   The CBC shows an elevated WBC count (leukocytosis) with a slight decrease in the percentage of neutrophils (segs; neutropenia). The percentage of lymphocytes is increased (lymphocytosis). No atypical lymphocytes were noted on the peripheral blood smear. RBC counts, parameters, and the platelet count are all normal.

2. **What is the significance of the above findings in regards to the patient's symptoms?**

   The most likely explanation for the WBC picture above is a viral infection. Acute viral illness may raise or lower the total WBC count. More specific is the finding of lymphocytosis – this is a typical body response to viral infection. The absence of atypical lymphocytes on the peripheral smear makes infectious mononucleosis less likely, but does not, by itself, exclude the possibility.

3. **Does the CBC suggest that the patient might be dehydrated?**

   No – evidence of hemoconcentration (elevation of RBC, WBC, and platelet counts) is not present. However, the *absence* of a finding, such as hemoconcentration, is usually less helpful than if it was present (and supported the diagnosis of dehydration). So, even though the CBC is not compatible with dehydration, it's still possible that the patient is dehydrated – this wouldn't be real surprising, considering the clinical history, would it?

4. **If the patient is dehydrated, what other lab tests might help support the diagnosis? What would you expect to find?**

   Two types of tests might be helpful, the UA and the Chemistry Panel:

   - UA – increased urine specific gravity; ketones present on dipstick
   - Chemistry Panel – increased sodium, BUN, Cr; BUN/Cr ratio > 10

   The UA, shown on the next page, is compatible with dehydration – the specific gravity is significantly elevated and 2+ ketones are present:

Camp Rothenberg Infirmary
Urinalysis (UA)

TEST	PATIENT	NORMAL
Color	dk yellow	Pale yellow to amber
Appearance	cloudy	Clear to slightly hazy
SG	1.030	1.015-1.025
pH	5.0	4.5-8.0
Glucose	-	Negative
Ketones	++	Negative
Blood	-	Negative
Protein	-	Negative
Bilirubin	-	Negative
Urobilinogen	-	Negative-trace
Nitrate	-	Negative
Leuk Est.	-	Negative
Casts	-	Negative
RBC	-	Rare or negative
WBC	-	Negative or rare
Crystals	-	Negative
Epithelial	-	Few
Bacteria	-	None

Now, let's look at the Chemistry Panel and see if the findings there also support the diagnosis of dehydration (think about what you'd expect to find):

Camp Rothenberg Infirmary
Chemistry Panel

TEST	PATIENT	NORMAL
Na^+	150	135-145 mEq/L
K^+	4.6	3.5-5.3 mEq/L
Cl^-	108	98-106 mEq/L
HCO_3^-	35	23-30 mmol/L
BS	109	65-110 mg/dl
BUN	30	7-18 mg/dl
Cr	1.7	0.6-1.3 mg/dl

QUESTIONS

1. What are the lab findings?
2. Do the above findings support the diagnosis of dehydration?
3. Are there other possible explanations for the bicarbonate level, besides dehydration?
4. Considering the patient's clinical history and the available lab work, what is the most likely "working diagnosis?"

1. **What are the lab findings?**

On the Chemistry Panel, all the values, except for the blood sugar (BS), are elevated.

2. **Do the above findings support the diagnosis of dehydration?**

Yes – uniform or near-uniform (the case here) elevation or decrease of test values on a given panel (that measures *concentrations*) suggests that fluids (either dehydration or overhydration) are the most likely cause. Always think of "fluids and drugs" early in the differential diagnosis of any laboratory abnormalities.

Sodium is the most sensitive of the electrolytes to fluid balance. It is often elevated in dehydration when the remainder of the parameters (except BUN/Cr, of course) remain normal. Elevation of the BUN and Cr, as well as the BUN/Cr ratio > 10, also support the diagnosis of dehydration.

3. **Are there other possible explanations for the bicarbonate level, besides dehydration?**

The elevated bicarbonate level indicates the presence of a metabolic alkalosis. Hemoconcentration (dehydration) may be responsible for a portion of this elevation. Loss of stomach acid via vomiting and subsequent metabolic alkalosis (with elevation of the bicarbonate level) is likely also present.

4. **Considering the patient's clinical history and the available lab work, what is the most likely "working diagnosis?"**

The most likely explanation for the entire constellation of findings present in this patient is viral gastroenteritis with moderate dehydration. Clinically, I've found that simply replenishing fluid volume with 1-2 liters of normal saline IV over 1-2 hours leads to remarkable improvement in most patients. Rarely, do they require antiemetics.

CASE 20

48 year old male involved in a motor vehicle accident (MVA); MediAlert® tag partially destroyed – the readable portion says "heart valve." No significant injuries are noted on the patient's physical exam.

Camp Rothenberg Infirmary
"Incomplete" Blood Cell Count (CBC)

PARAMETER	PATIENT RESULT	NORMAL RANGE
Hb g/dl	15	M 14.0-17.4 F 12.0-16.0
Hct (%)	45	M 36-48 F 42-52
MCV (fl)	nl	84-96
MCH pg	nl	28-34
MCHC g/dl	nl	32-36
Plts X 10^3	150	140-400

Camp Rothenberg Infirmary
Coagulation Profile

Test	Patient	Normal range
Protime (PT)	35	11.0-13.0 seconds
International normalized ratio (INR)	4.0	1.0 - 1.5
Partial thromboplastin time (PTT)	35	30-45 seconds

QUESTIONS

1. What are the lab findings?
2. What is the significance of the Coagulation Profile results?
3. At this point, is there any need to make changes in either the patient's oral anticoagulation regimen or to otherwise alter the PT/INR (e.g., vitamin K, fresh frozen plasma)?

ANSWERS

1. What are the lab findings?

RBC count and parameters, as well as the platelet count are WNL. Though not given in the above example, the WBC count and differential were also normal. The PTT is normal, but both the PT and INR are elevated. [**NOTE**: many laboratories now only report the INR, not both INR and PT; both are shown in these case studies for your reference.]

2. What is the significance of the Coagulation Profile results?

The PT/INR results would be bothersome in a patient who was not taking oral anticoagulants. Though most of the patient's MediAlert® tag is damaged, the words "heart valve," combined with the PT/INR values here suggest that he is on oral anticoagulants. This fact was confirmed by the patient – since his aortic valve replacement surgery (placement of a Bjork-Shiley tilting disc artificial valve) five years ago, he's been on warfarin (Coumadin®), 5 mg daily. His last INR, one month ago, was 4.0.

The PT of 35 is higher than most clinicians like, even for a patient with a mechanical cardiac valve. When PT was used, instead of INR, most providers tried to keep the PT in the range of 23-25 for these patients. Unfortunately, the drawback of the PT test is that normals vary from lab to lab, and even in the same lab, when different kits (containing various types of thromboplastin) were used. The beauty of the INR is that a standardized thromboplastin is used for reference. Thus, the INR is reproducible and "believable" just about everywhere.

3. At this point, is there any need to make changes in either the patient's oral anticoagulation regimen or to otherwise alter the PT/INR (e.g., vitamin K, fresh frozen plasma)?

The preferred INR range for patients with artificial heart valves is 3.0 - 4.5. In light of the life-threatening problems that could occur with inadequate anticoagulation (clotting and occlusion of the valve), I think it's probably best in this patient to use the INR, not the PT, and make no changes in the levels of anticoagulation. However, this conclusion is based on just the information we currently have. The results of the patient's UA just came back from the lab. Let's see how they fit in . . .

Camp Rothenberg Infirmary
Urinalysis (UA)

PARAMETER	PATIENT RESULT	NORMAL RANGE
Color	yellow	Pale yellow to amber
Appearance	clr	Clear to slightly hazy
Specific gravity	1.020	1.015-1.025
pH	6.5	4.5-8.0
Glucose	-	Negative
Ketones	-	Negative
Blood	+++	Negative
Protein	+	Negative
Bilirubin	-	Negative
Urobilinogen	-	Negative-trace
Nitrate for bacteria	-	Negative
Leucocyte esterase	-	Negative
Casts	-	Negative
RBC	++ (30 RBC/HPF)	Rare or negative
WBC	-	Negative or rare
Crystals	-	Negative
Epithelial cells	few	Few
Bacteria	-	None

QUESTIONS

1. What are the lab findings?
2. In light of the patient's history, what is the significance of the above findings?
3. What further tests are necessary?

ANSWERS

1. **What are the lab findings?**

The dipstick is 3+ positive for blood; on microscopic examination, ~ 30 RBC per high powered field (HPF) were noted.

2. **In light of the patient's history, what is the significance of the above findings?**

Hematuria following trauma suggests injury to some part of the urinary system. The presence of intact RBCs on microscopic exam suggests, but does not prove, kidney trauma. Therapeutic levels of oral anticoagulation do *not* result in hematuria – when this is present, you should always look for a second lesion. In this patient, urinary tract trauma is the most likely culprit. In a nontrauma situation, the most common offender is an occult tumor of the urinary tract.

3. **What further tests are necessary?**

Current recommendations state that if there are less than 40-50 RBC/HPF on microscopic examination of the urine, further diagnostic tests are unlikely to be helpful. Simple observation is suggested. The confounder in this particular situation is the fact that the patient is on anticoagulants. Conceivably, this could worsen bleeding from a relatively minor renal contusion. For this reason, the patient's caregivers chose to obtain a contrast CT scan of the kidneys and abdomen – it showed a small right renal contusion, with no evidence of active bleeding or significant subcapsular hematoma. The patient was observed in the hospital for 24 hours – there were no changes in his symptoms (he remained asymptomatic), vital signs (they remained stable), or the CBC (remained normal). Repeat CT scan, done as an outpatient three days later, showed complete resolution of the renal contusion. The patient was kept on his same dose of Coumadin®.

CASE 21

56 year old female -- strong odor of alcohol; somewhat lethargic and uncooperative.

Camp Rothenberg Infirmary
Complete Blood Cell Count (CBC)

PARAMETER	PATIENT RESULT	NORMAL RANGE
WBC X 10^3	4.5	5.0-10.0
%Band	0	1-3
%Seg	30	50-62
%Eosin	0	1-4
%Baso	0	0-1
%Mono	0	0-5
%Lymph	70	25-45
RBC X 10^6	3.0	4.5-5.5
Hb g/dl	10.0	M 14.0-17.4 F 12.0-16.0
Hct (%)	30.0	M 36-48 F 42-52
MCV (fl)	nl	84-96
MCH pg	nl	28-34
MCHC g/dl	nl	32-36
Plts X 10^3	100,000	140-400

QUESTIONS

1. What are the lab findings?
2. What are some potential causes of the above WBC picture?
3. Regarding the RBC count, what general condition is present?
4. Describe how you would further classify the above condition.
5. What are possible causes of this condition in the above patient?
6. What are possible explanations for the platelet count?

246

ANSWERS

1.   What are the lab findings?

The WBC count is low (leukopenia) with a decreased percentage of segs (neutrophils; neutropenia) and an elevated percentage of lymphocytes (lymphocytosis). The RBC and H/H are low (anemia) with a normal MCV, MCH, and MCHC. The platelet count is moderately low (thrombocytopenia).

2.   What are some potential causes of the above WBC picture?

Leukopenia with lymphocytosis suggests, but does not prove, a viral infection. Another possible explanation is bone marrow suppression due to any cause. A potentially bothersome finding is that the total number of neutrophils is significantly decreased – 30% of 4500 = 1350 total neutrophils. Increased susceptibility to bacterial infections starts to become an issue when the total neutrophil count falls below 1000, however, the risk is greatest when the number is below 500 cells. Realistically, this is probably not a concern in this patient, at this time. A final consideration here is hemodilution.

3.   Regarding the RBC count, what general condition is present?

The above findings suggest anemia (decreased numbers of RBCs). We can further classify the type of anemia present, as discussed in the next question.

4.   Describe how you would further classify the above condition.

To classify anemias, we determine whether the cells are "ugly" or not – in other words, are they normal sized, too big, or too small? The easiest way to do this is to look at the MCV, a direct reflection of cell size. In this case, the MCV is normal, so the red cells are normal in size. This is termed a normocytic anemia. Normal red cell size suggests that the "intrinsic machinery" of the cell is intact. However, the bone marrow simply isn't making enough of these *normal cells* to keep up with the demand – and the patient becomes anemic.

5.   What are possible causes of this condition in the above patient?

The most common causes of normocytic anemia are chronic disease or acute bleeding. At this point, we have no information that helps point us in a particular diagnostic direction.

6.   What are possible explanations for the platelet count?

Overhydration, with dilution of all CBC parameters is a possible explanation, but should not change the relative percentages of segs and lymphocytes. Bone marrow suppression from any cause could easily explain the entire CBC picture.

PARAMETER	PATIENT RESULT	NORMAL RANGE
Color	orange-brown	Pale yellow to amber
Appearance	cloudy	Clear to slightly hazy
Specific gravity	1.027	1.015-1.025
pH	7.0	4.5-8.0
Glucose	-	Negative
Ketones	+++	Negative
Blood	-	Negative
Protein	-	Negative
Bilirubin	++	Negative
Urobilinogen	tr	Negative-trace
Nitrate for bacteria	-	Negative
Leucocyte esterase	-	Negative
Casts	-	Negative
RBC	-	Rare or negative
WBC	-	Negative or rare
Crystals	-	Negative
Epithelial cells	-	Few
Bacteria	-	None

QUESTIONS

1. What are the lab findings?
2. What additional diagnostic information does the UA add to the picture?
3. Summarize what we know to this point, both clinically and lab-wise, about this patient.
4. What other lab tests would be of interest to you at this point?

ANSWERS

1. What are the lab findings?

The urine color is abnormal and the specific gravity is increased. The dipstick is positive for ketones (3+), bilirubin (++), and urobilinogen (tr). The microscopic exam is normal.

2. What additional diagnostic information does the UA add to the picture?

The UA suggests that the patient is somewhat dehydrated (increased specific gravity, ketonuria). There are, however, alternative explanations (read on . . .). In addition, bilirubinuria suggests a problem with the patient's hepatobiliary system – the fact that there is a small amount of urobilinogen present in the urine, a normal finding, rules out complete hepatobiliary obstruction. Of course, partial obstruction and/or hepatocellular injury are still possibilities.

3. Summarize what we know to this point, both clinically and lab-wise, about this patient.

Thus far, we know the following information:

- The patient smells of alcohol and has an abnormal mental status.
- She has a WBC that suggests either viral illness or bone marrow suppression.
- She has a normocytic anemia and a moderately depressed platelet count.
- She is likely dehydrated, at least based on the urine specific gravity elevation and the presence of 3+ ketonuria.
- She has some type of hepatobiliary disorder – complete obstruction is extremely unlikely.

4. What other lab tests would be of interest to you at this point?

I'd be interested in seeing the results of the patient's Liver Panel, Coagulation Profile, and Chemistry Profile. For those of you who are, appropriately, wondering about the blood alcohol level and the toxicology screen results, you'll have to wait a little bit longer   the lab just told me that they are "pending!"

Parameter	Patient result	Normal value (adults)
Albumin	2.1	3.8-5.0 g/dl
Ammonia (NH$_4$)	45	9-33 umol/L
Bilirubin, total	4.0	0.2-1.0 mg/dl
Bilirubin, direct (conjugated)	3.7	0.0-0.2 mg/dl
Bilirubin, indirect (unconjugated)	0.3	0.2-0.8 mg/dl
Alanine transaminase (ALT, SGPT [serum glutamic-pyruvic transaminase])	150	7-56 U/L
Alkaline phosphatase (ALP)	180	17-142 IU/L
Aspartate transaminase (AST; serum glutamic-oxaloacetic transaminase [SGOT])	60	5-40 U/L
Gamma-glutamyltransferase (GGT)	300	5-85 U/L (males); 5-55 U/L (females)
Lactic acid dehydrogenase (LDH)	650	313-618 U/L
Total protein	3	6.0-8.0 g/dl

QUESTIONS

1. What are the lab findings?
2. What is the significance of the bilirubin levels?
3. What is the significance of the enzyme (ALT[SGPT], AST [SGOT], alkaline phosphatase [alk phos]) levels?
4. What information does the gamma-glutamyltransferase (GGT) level add to the picture?
5. What information does the lactic acid dehydrogenase (LDH) level add to the picture?
6. What is the significance of the ammonia level?
7. What is the significance of the albumin and total protein levels?
8. In light of the above findings, what can we conclude regarding the patient's overall liver function?
9. Assuming our conclusion above (question #8) is correct, what would you predict the Coagulation Profile to show?
10. By the way, the blood alcohol and toxicology screen results are back . . .

ANSWERS

1.   What are the lab findings?

Albumin and total protein levels are low. The remainder of the parameters are elevated.

2.   What is the significance of the bilirubin levels?

The total bilirubin is elevated, with a preponderance of conjugated bilirubin. This explains the bilirubinuria. Sometimes patients with elevated bilirubin levels do not demonstrate clinical jaundice – a common reason for this is that we typically examine them in rooms with fluorescent lighting. Rarely will clinical jaundice, especially if low-grade, be evident under these conditions. Jaundice (especially scleral icterus) is best seen in natural sunlight (bring the patient by the window). Due to the patient's altered mental status, this could not be done during the initial evaluation – when she was stabilized, repeat exam did reveal 2+ scleral icterus.

3.   What is the significance of the enzyme (ALT[SGPT], AST [SGOT], alkaline phosphatase [alk phos]) levels?

The alk phos elevation is minimal and is not very helpful – in a 56-year old woman, mild elevations of alk phos could occur from bone disease, such as osteoporosis, Paget's disease, or tumor metastases (most likely from breast cancer). Elevations of the ALT/AST (SGPT/SGOT) levels, however, are relatively liver specific. Though the ALT (SGPT) level is greater than twice normal, the AST (SGOT) level is not. These elevations, taken together, are compatible with either hepatocellular injury or partial obstruction. There is another explanation for the relatively low levels of liver enzymes noted in this patient – give it some thought, and I'll tell you the answer in #8, below.

4.   What information does the gamma-glutamyltransferase (GGT) level add to the picture?

Once the patient has clinical symptoms of liver disease (e.g., jaundice), the GGT becomes noncontributory, with one exception (read on . . .). This test is most helpful as an early screening test to implicate liver disease (of any type – hepatocellular damage *or* obstruction) when all else is normal. Once all the other parameters on the Liver Panel are abnormal and/or there is clinical jaundice present, the GGT doesn't really tell you much more than you should have already concluded – the patient has hepatobiliary disease. The only exception to this is if a patient is jaundiced due to excess unconjugated bilirubin (e.g., hemolytic anemia, congenital conjugation defect) – a normal GGT here may help rule out liver disease. The reason the GGT is included in the present patient is because it comes routinely as part of the Camp Rothenberg Infirmary Liver Profile – and, it is cheaper to get the entire profile, rather than order selected tests individually.

251

5. **What information does the lactic acid dehydrogenase (LDH) level add to the picture?**

Many laboratories no longer routinely include the LDH level as part of a Liver Panel. LDH elevations are fairly nonspecific and may arise from hemolytic anemia, or diseases of the liver, heart, skeletal muscle, lung, or brain. In this case, I included it just to make certain that you are aware of its' relatively limited value under most circumstances, including those of the present patient.

6. **What is the significance of the ammonia level?**

The liver is responsible for metabolism of ammonia waste products to urea. Ammonia is generated in the gastrointestinal (GI) tract, then absorbed through the portal vein, and removed by the liver. The relationship between elevated ammonia levels and liver disease has been recognized for many years. Increased ammonia levels are associated with fulminant hepatic failure, Reye's syndrome, cirrhosis, GI bleeding, and portal-systemic shunting of blood.

7. **What is the significance of the albumin and total protein levels?**

Low levels of albumin and total protein can occur as a result of poor nutrition, severe liver disease (loss of synthetic function), or a combination.

8. **In light of the above findings, what can we conclude regarding the patient's overall liver function?**

Unless the patient has concomitant GI bleeding to explain the ammonia level, the most likely conclusion here is that she has significant hepatic failure. This would explain her mental status, as well as most of the laboratory abnormalities we've seen so far. An interesting lab feature of liver failure is that the worse it gets, the less likely are significant elevations of ALT/AST (SGPT/SGOT) to occur. The reason is that so many hepatocytes have been destroyed already, there is less residual enzyme to be released into the blood when more are injured. This may explain why the current patient's enzyme levels are only mildly elevated.

9. **Assuming our conclusion above (question #8) is correct, what would you predict the Coagulation Profile to show?**

The liver is responsible for synthesis of clotting factors II, VII, IX, and X – these are the parameters measured by either the PT or INR tests. I'd expect the PT/INR to be elevated, as if the patient was on oral anticoagulants. As with the albumin and total protein levels, abnormal coagulation tests in liver failure are an indication of loss of synthetic functions. The PTT should be relatively unaffected.

10. By the way, the blood alcohol and toxicology screen results are back . . .

Both are negative – this suggests that the patient's altered mental status is not due to either drug or alcohol intoxication. The "odor of alcohol" on her breath could be due to a number of reasons. Patients with liver often have a funny breath odor, fetor hepaticus – a musty, sweet odor that is sometimes mistaken for alcohol. Chemically, this odor is due to the formation of mercaptans – a group of sulfur-containing organic chemical substances. The body produces them naturally during digestion of beer, garlic, and some other foods. They are normally excreted by the liver.

The negative alcohol and toxicology results in this patient emphasize the value of these tests as medical tests (see Chapter 12, Other Tests (Drug and Alcohol Screening). Despite ones' initial temptation to assume the patient is simply drunk (odor of "alcohol", altered mental status), these tests effectively exclude that possibility. Combined with the results of the patient's other tests, it's clear that her "intoxication" is more likely due to hepatic wastes.

Let's see if the results of the Coagulation Profile matched our expectations:

Camp Rothenberg Infirmary
Coagulation Profile

Test	Patient	Normal range
Protime (PT)	16/12	11.0-13.0 seconds
International normalized ratio (INR)	2.5	1.0 - 1.5
Partial thromboplastin time (PTT)	40	30-45 seconds

As predicted, the PT and INR are elevated, suggesting impaired hepatic synthesis of factors II, VI, IX, and X. The PTT does not reflect the levels of these factors, so it often remains normal, even in severe liver failure. The remaining test we indicated an interest in earlier was the Chemistry Panel. The results are shown on the next page.

Test	Patient result	Normal value (adult)
Sodium (Na^+)	125	135-145 mEq/L
Potassium (K^+)	3.5	3.5-5.3 mEq/L
Chloride (Cl^-)	95	98-106 mEq/L
Bicarbonate (HCO_3^-)	28	23-30 mmol/L
Calcium (Ca^{2+})	6.2	8.6-10.0 mg/dl
Magnesium (Mg^{2+})	1.3	1.3-2.1 mEq/L
Blood sugar (BS)	60	65-110 mg/dl
Blood urea nitrogen (BUN)	5.1	7-18 mg/dl
Creatinine (Cr)	0.5	0.6-1.3 mg/dl

QUESTIONS

1. What are the lab findings?
2. What is the significance of the sodium and chloride levels?
3. What is the significance of the calcium and magnesium levels?
4. What is the significance of the blood sugar level?
5. What is the significance of the BUN/Cr levels?
6. Summarize what we know to this point, both clinically and lab-wise, about this patient.
7. Generally speaking, what are the most likely diagnostic possibilities?
8. Are there other tests that may reveal a specific diagnosis?

1.   **What are the lab findings?**

The following parameters are decreased: sodium, chloride, calcium, magnesium, blood sugar, BUN, creatinine (Cr).

2.   **What is the significance of the sodium and chloride levels?**

The most common cause of hyponatremia (and accompanying hypochloremia, which sometimes occurs) is dilutional (fluid retention). In liver disease, there is sometimes overstimulation of antidiuretic hormone (ADH) – this leads to hyponatremia. Whether this is the case here is difficult to say, though it is a possibility. The increased urine specific gravity could be caused by ADH secretion leading to fluid retention by the kidneys. This would also cause dilutional decreases in sodium and chloride. In fact, significant hemodilution could decrease many of the measured lab values. Remember, in any laboratory abnormality, always consider fluids and drugs first!

3.   **What is the significance of the calcium and magnesium levels?**

Hemodilution could explain some of the changes – however, both calcium and magnesium (as measured on standard Chemistry Panels) are protein bound. So a decrease in the serum albumin level (for any reason) may lead to a decrease in the measured calcium and magnesium levels.

4.   **What is the significance of the blood sugar level?**

Hemodilution or hemoconcentration may affect the blood sugar level, but clinically significant changes for either of these reasons are unusual. I'd bet that the most likely cause is a combination of the patient's liver disease and poor nutrition. Recall, the liver is the main site for storage of glucose, in the form of glycogen. In addition, the liver normally contributes to glucose metabolism by manufacturing new glucose – gluconeogenesis. Both the ability to break down glycogen (glycogenolysis) and to gluconeogenesis are impaired in moderate to severe liver disease.

5.   **What is the significance of the BUN/Cr levels?**

Hemoconcentration is a common cause of elevations in the BUN and Cr, often with a BUN/Cr ratio > 10. Hemodilution has less predictable effects on the BUN and Cr. Though this remains a possibility in our patient, a more likely explanation for depressed levels of BUN and Cr is a combination of poor nutrition and liver disease. The liver normally metabolizes ammonia waste products to urea, most of which is then excreted in the urine. A small amount is normally found in the blood – this is what is measured in the laboratory as blood urea nitrogen (BUN). Poor nutrition can lead to decreased protein intake and reduce the BUN and Cr levels (creatinine reflects muscle mass and muscle breakdown). Hepatic dysfunction (as is present in the current patient) prevents adequate metabolism of ammonia (thus, the increased serum ammonia level), so less urea is formed. As a result, the BUN goes down. The two major causes of low BUN are poor diet and liver disease. Both are likely operative in our patient here.

6. **Summarize what we know to this point, both clinically and lab-wise, about this patient.**

Thus far, we know the following information:

- The patient smells of alcohol and has an abnormal mental status. Based on the negative blood alcohol and toxicology screens, intoxication is not a part of the problem.
- She has a WBC that suggests either viral illness or bone marrow suppression.
- She has a normocytic anemia and a moderately depressed platelet count.
- She may be dehydrated – alternatively, the high urine specific gravity could be due to secretion of ADH as a result of the liver disease. The resulting hemodilution may contribute to low levels of several different measured parameters. ADH secretion should *not*, however, lead to an *increase* in the urine ketones.
- She has some type of hepatobiliary disorder – complete obstruction is extremely unlikely.
- She likely has severe liver dysfunction, as manifested by decreased synthetic function (low albumin/protein, low glucose, abnormal PT/INR), low BUN/Cr, and elevated ammonia levels).
- Her nutritional status is poor (low glucose, calcium, magnesium, BUN/Cr). These findings are likely secondary to a combination of hepatic dysfunction and poor nutrition.

7. **Generally speaking, what are the most likely diagnostic possibilities?**

All in all, this unfortunate lady is a "metabolic mess." In a complex patient such as this, one general principle is often helpful – if all or most of the picture can be explained by a *single entity*, then that entity is the most likely diagnostic possible. This isn't always the case, but why invoke multiple causes when one will explain all or most of the situation?

The most logical explanation for the overall picture, clinical and lab-wise, is moderately severe liver disease. The resultant hemodilution explains at least a portion of decreased levels in many of the measured parameters – ADH secretion caused the increased urine specific gravity. The ketonuria (3+) remains elusive – in fact, the patient's caregivers didn't think this made sense either. When they repeated the dipstick UA, no ketones were noted. Apparently, there was a bad batch of chemical dipsticks – these were replaced quickly.

Chronic liver disease has a suppressive effect on the bone marrow, leading to the CBC findings. The Liver Panel findings are compatible with hepatocellular injury and combined with the albumin, protein, and ammonia results, as well as the Coagulation Profile, suggest moderate to severe liver failure. For the reasons discussed in the previous questions of this section, the Chemistry Panel results are also easily explained by liver failure.

8. **Are there other tests that may reveal a specific diagnosis?**

Yes. One potential cause of the patient's liver problems is primary biliary cirrhosis (PBC). About 90% of patients with PBC have autoantibodies against specific mitochondrial proteins (the E2 subunits of the oxo-acid dehydrogenase complexes). Approximately 50% of patients have antinuclear antibodies, sometimes against very specific proteins (nuclear pore membrane protein gp210, transcriptional activator Sp100, inner nuclear membrane protein LBR). In addition, IgM levels and cholesterol are often elevated. Various hepatitis antigen and antibody measurements may also be helpful in finding other diagnoses. In PBC, as well as in several other liver diseases (e.g., alcoholic cirrhosis, chronic hepatitis) histological examination of liver tissue is of central diagnostic importance. Thus, a liver biopsy is often necessary to finalize a diagnosis. Prior to performing the biopsy, the patient's caretakers would need to carefully assess the risk:benefit ratio, especially in light of the abnormal PT and INR.

REFERENCES

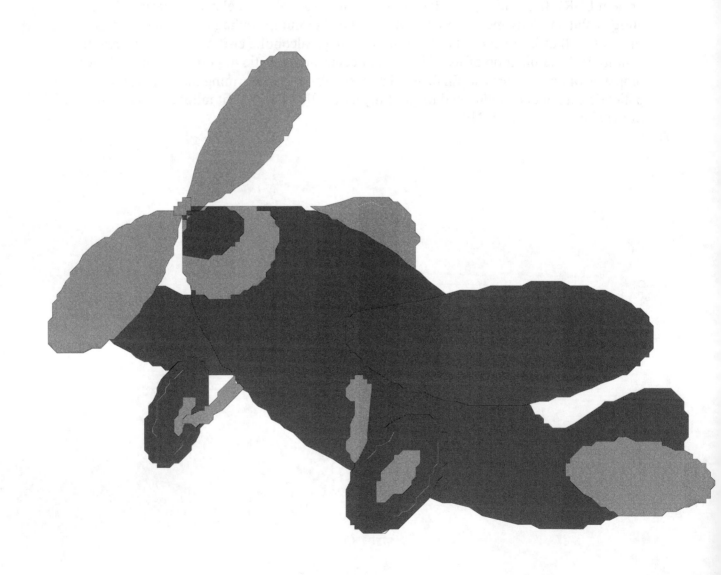

REFERENCES

1.   Adapted, with permission, from: M.A. Rothenberg, Pathophysiology: A Plain English Approach, PESI Health Care (Eau Claire), [C] Mikel A. Rothenberg, M.D., 2001.

2.   N. Deka, et al., *Isolation of the novel agent from human stool samples that is associated with sporadic non-A, non-B hepatitis*, 68 J Virol 7810-5 (1994).

3.   M. Tacke, et al., *Humoral immune response to the E2 protein of hepatitis G virus is associated with long-term recovery from infection and reveals a high frequency of hepatitis G virus exposure among healthy blood donors*, 26 Hepatology 1626 (1997).

4.   E. Tanaka, et al., *Evolution of hepatitis G virus infection and antibody response to envelope protein in patients with transfusion-associated non-A, non-B hepatitis*, 5 J Viral Hep 153 (1998).

5.   Panel on Clinical Practices for Treatment of HIV Infection convened by the Department of Health and Human Services (DHHS), *Guidelines for the Use of Antiretroviral Agents in HIV-1-Infected Adults and Adolescents*, October 29, 2004, http://www.aidsinfo.nih.gov/guidelines/adult/AA_102904.html, accessed 12/19/04.

6.   G.R. Kaufmann, et al., *CD4 T-lymphocyte recovery in individuals with advanced HIV-1 infection receiving potent antiretroviral therapy for 4 years: the Swiss HIV Cohort Study*, 163 Arch Intern Med 2187-95 (2003).

7.   J.W. Mellors, et al., *Quantitation of HIV-1 RNA in Plasma Predicts Outcome after Seroconversion*, 122 Ann Intern Med 573-9 (April 1995).

8.   Panel on Clinical Practices for Treatment of HIV Infection convened by the Department of Health and Human Services (DHHS), *Guidelines for the Use of Antiretroviral Agents in HIV-1-Infected Adults and Adolescents*, October 29, 2004, http://www.aidsinfo.nih.gov/guidelines/adult/AA_102904.html, accessed 12/19/04.

9.   Panel on Clinical Practices for Treatment of HIV Infection convened by the Department of Health and Human Services (DHHS), *Guidelines for the Use of Antiretroviral Agents in HIV-1-Infected Adults and Adolescents*, October 29, 2004, http://www.aidsinfo.nih.gov/guidelines/adult/AA_102904.html, accessed 12/19/04.

10.   J.A. Bartlett, et al., *Overview of the effectiveness of triple combination therapy in antiretroviral-naïve HIV-1 infected adults*, 15 AIDS 1369-77 (2001).

11.   G.J. Weverling, et al., *Alternative multidrug regimen provides improved suppression of HIV-1 replication over triple therapy*, 12 AIDS 117-22 (1998).

12.   J.A. DeSimone, et al., *Inflammatory reactions in HIV-1-infected persons after initiation of highly active antiretroviral therapy*, 133 Ann Intern Med 447-54 (2000).

13.   B. Ledergerber, et al., *Clinical progression and virological failure on highly active antiretroviral therapy in HIV-1 patients: A prospective cohort study. Swiss HIV Cohort Study*, 353 Lancet 863-8 (1999).

14.   S. Grabar, et al., *Clinical outcome of patients with HIV-1 infection according to immunologic and virologic response after 6 months of highly active antiretroviral therapy*, 133 Ann Intern Med 401-10 (2002).

15.   Adapted, with permission, from: M.A. Rothenberg, Pathophysiology: A Plain English Approach, PESI Health Care (Eau Claire), [C] Mikel A. Rothenberg, M.D., 2001.

16.   O. Nagagawa, et al., *Rapid transcriptional activation and early mRNA turnover of BNP in cardiocyte hypertrophy: evidence for BNP as an "emergency" cardiac hormone against ventricular overload*, 96 J Clin Invest 1280-7 (1995); K. Maeda, et al., *Plasma brain natriuretic peptide as a biochemical marker of high left ventricular end-diastolic pressure in patients with symptomatic left ventricular dysfunction*, 135 Am Heart J 825-32 (1998).

17.   D.J. Campbell, et al., *Prediction of Heart Failure by Amino Terminal-pro-B-Type Natriuretic Peptide and C-Reactive Protein in Subjects With Cerebrovascular Disease*, Hypertension, Nov 2004; 10.1161/01.HYP.0000151103.02424.c3.

18.   E.A. Ramoska, et. al., *Reliability of patient history in determining the possibility of pregnancy*, 18 Ann Emerg Med 48-50 (January 1989).

19.   L.A. Boutiette and G.V. Anderson, *Heteropic Pregnancy*, 7 J Emerg Med 33-5 (1989).

20.   National Cholesterol Education Program, *Third Report of the Expert Panel on Detection, Evaluation, and Treatment of High Blood Cholesterol in Adults (Adult Treatment Panel III) Full Report*, NIH Publication 02-5215, September 2002, http://www.nhlbi.nih.gov/guidelines/cholesterol/atp3full.pdf, accessed 9/26/04.

21.   National Cholesterol Education Program, *Third Report of the Expert Panel on Detection, Evaluation, and Treatment of High Blood Cholesterol in Adults (Adult Treatment Panel III) Executive Summary*, NIH Publication 01-3760, May 2001, http://www.nhlbi.nih.gov/guidelines/cholesterol/atp3xsum.pdf, accessed 9/26/04. Also published in: 285 JAMA 2486-2497 (2001).

22.   E. Stein, et al., *Achieving lipoprotein goals in patients at high risk with severe hypercholesterolemia: Efficacy and safety of ezetimibe co-administered with atorvastatin*, 148 Am Heart J 447-55 (Sep 2004); L. Simons, et al., *Effects of ezetimibe added to on-going statin therapy on the lipid profile of hypercholesterolemic patients with diabetes mellitus or metabolic syndrome*, 20 Curr Med Res Opin 1437-45 (Sep 2004); J. Jurado, et al., *Effectiveness of ezetimibe in clinical practice*, 93 Am J Cardiol

641-3 (Mar 2004); C.A. Dujovne, et al., *Efficacy and safety of a potent new selective cholesterol absorption inhibitor, ezetimibe, in patients with primary hypercholesterolemia*, 90 Am J Cardiol 1092-7 (Nov 2002).

23.   B.A. Griffin, *Low-density lipoprotein heterogeneity*, 9 Bailliere Clin Endocrinol Metabol 687-703 (1995).

24.   R.M. Krauss, et al., *Lipoprotein subclasses in genetic studies: the Berkeley data* , 10 Genet Epidemiol 523-8 (1993).

25.   R.M. Krauss, *Heterogeneity of plasma low-density lipoproteins and atherosclerosis risk*, 5 Curr Opin Lipidol 339-49 (1994).

26.   T. O'Brien and T.T. Nguyen, *Lipids and lipoproteins in women*, 72 Mayo Clin Proc 235-44 (1997).

27.   Y. Bosse, et al., *Genetics of LDL particle heterogeneity: from genetic epidemiology to DNA-based variations*, 45 J Lipid Res 1008-26 (Jun 2004).

28.   B. Lamarche, et al., *Fasting Insulin and Apolipoprotein B Levels and Low-Density Lipoprotein Particle Size as Risk Factors for Ischemic Heart Disease*, 279 Jour Am Med Assoc 1955-61 (1998).

29.   N. Barzilai, *Unique Lipoprotein Phenotype and Genotype Associated With Exceptional Longevity*, 290 JAMA 2030-40 (2003).

30.   I. Rajman, et al., *Particle size: the key to the atherogenic lipoprotein?* 12 QJM 708-20 (1994).

31.   B. Lamarche, et al., *Small, Dense Low-Density Lipoprotein Particles as a Predictor of the Risk of Ischemic Heart Disease in Men. Prospective Results From the Quebec Cardiovascular Study*, 95 Circulation 69-75 (1997).

32.   See, for example: http://www.atherotech.com/content/images/presskit/factsheet.htm (Press release); http://www.4qc.com/products/lipoprint/faq_prof.html (Company web site with references).

33.   J.F. Mauger, et al., *Effect of different forms of dietary hydrogenated fats on LDL particle size*, 78 Am. J. Clinical Nutrition 370 (2003).

34.   T.A. Mori, et al., *Purified eicosapentaenoic and docosahexaenoic acids have differential effects on serum lipids and lipoproteins, LDL particle size, glucose, and insulin in mildly hyperlipidemic men*, 71 Am J Clin Nutr 1085-94 (2000).

35.   J.M. McKenney, et al., *Effect of niacin and atorvastatin on lipoprotein subclasses in patients with atherogenic dyslipidemia*, 88 Am J Cardiol 270-4 (Aug 2001).

36.   National Cholesterol Education Program, *Information About the Update of the Adult Treatment Panel III Guidelines*, http://www.nhlbi.nih.gov/guidelines/cholesterol/upd-info_prof.htm, accessed 9/26/04. Also published in: 110 Circulation 227-39 (2004).

37.   P.T. Sager, et al., *Effect of coadministration of ezetimibe and simvastatin on high-sensitivity C-reactive protein*, 92 Am J Cardiol 1414-8 (Dec 2003).

38.   M.A. van de Ree, et al., *Strong decrease of high sensitivity C-reactive protein with high-dose atorvastatin in patients with type 2 diabetes mellitus*, 166 Atherosclerosis 129-35 (Jan 2003).

39.   E. Chan, et al., *Effect of Atorvastatin and Fish Oil on Plasma High-Sensitivity C-Reactive Protein Concentrations in Individuals with Visceral Obesity*, 48 Clin. Chem. 877-83 (Jun 2002).

40.   I.T. Lee, et al., *Simvastatin reduces plasma concentration of high-sensitivity C-reactive protein in type 2 diabetic patients with hyperlipidemia*, 16 J Diabetes Complications 382-5 (Nov 2002).

41.   T.A. Pearson, et al., AHA/CDC *Scientific Statement – Markers of Inflammation and Cardiovascular Disease Application to Clinical and Public Health Practice: A Statement for Healthcare Professionals From the Centers for Disease Control and Prevention and the American Heart Association*, 107 Circulation 499 (2003).

42.   W. Koenig, *C-reactive protein and cardiovascular risk: Has the time come for screening the general population?* 47 Clinical Chemistry 9-10 (2001).

43.   L.M. Biasucci, et al., *Elevated levels of C-reactive protein at discharge in patients with unstable angina predict recurrent instability*, 99 Circulation 855-60 (1999); R.J. de Winter, et al., *Independent prognostic value of C-reactive protein and troponin I in patients with unstable angina or non-Q-wave myocardial infarction*, 42 Cardiovasc Res 240-5 (1999); E.R. Ferreiros, et al., *Independent prognostic value of elevated C-reactive protein in unstable angina*, 100 Circulation 1958-63 (1999).

44.   W.H. Yin, et al., *Independent prognostic value of elevated high-sensitivity C-reactive protein in chronic heart failure*, 147 Am Heart J 931-8 (May 2004).

45.   P.A. Clavien, et al., *Acute pancreatitis and normoamylasemia. Not an uncommon combination*, 210 Ann Surg 614-20 (1989).

46.   T. Takishima, et al., *Serum amylase level on admission in the diagnosis of blunt injury to the pancreas: its significance and limitations*, 226 Ann Surg 70-6 (1997).

47. Adapted from: National Cancer Institute, *Cancer Facts, The Prostate-Specific Antigen (PSA) Test: Questions and Answers*, 8/17/04, http://cis.nci.nih.gov/fact/5_29.htm, accessed 12/20/04.

48. I.M. Thompson, et al., *Prevalence of prostate cancer among men with a prostate-specific antigen level = 4.0 ng per milliliter*, 350 J Eng Jour Med 2239-46 (2004).

49. D.W. Keetch, et al., *Serial prostatic biopsies in men with persistently elevated serum prostate specific antigen values*, 151 J Urol 1571-4 (1994).

50. M.A. Blackwood and B.L. Weber, *BRCA1 and BRCA2: from molecular genetics to clinical medicine*, 16 J Clin Oncol 1969-77 (1998).

51. T.S. Frank, et al., *Sequence analysis of BRCA1 and BRCA2: correlation of mutations with family history and ovarian cancer risk*, 16 J Clin Oncol 2417-25 (1998).

52. Y. Miki, et al., *A strong candidate for the breast and ovarian cancer susceptibility gene BRCA1*, 266 Science 66-71 (1994); D. Ford, et al., *Risks of cancer in BRCA1-mutation carriers. Breast Cancer Linkage Consortium*, 343 Lancet 692-5 (1994).

53. *Cancer risks in BRCA2 mutation carriers. The Breast Cancer Linkage Consortium.* 91 J Natl Cancer Inst 1310-6 (1999).

54. D.J. Slamon, et al., *Studies of the HER-2/neu proto-oncogene in human breast and ovarian cancer*, 244 Science 707-12 (1989).

55. S. Shak, *Overview of the trastuzumab (Herceptin) anti-HER-2 monoclonal antibody clinical program in HER-2-overexpressing metastatic breast cancer. Herceptin Multinational Investigator Study Group*, 26 Semin Oncol 71-7 (Aug 1999).

56. S. Sjogren, et al., *Prognostic and predictive value of c-erbB-2 overexpression in primary breast cancer, alone and in combination with other prognostic markers*, 16 J Clin Oncol 462-9 (1998).

57. Herceptin® (Trastuzumab) full Prescribing Information; October 2003.

INDEX

271

293